BRINGING IT HOME

A Nurse's Story:
Life, Death, and In-Between in an Intensive Care Hospital

The Making of a Nurse

Lives in the Balance (editor)

Camp Nurse

Opening My Heart:
A Journey from Nurse to Patient and Back Again

Bringing It Home:
A Nurse Discovers Health Care Beyond the Hospital

BRINGING IT HOME

A NURSE DISCOVERS HEALTH CARE
BEYOND THE HOSPITAL

TILDA SHALOF

with JUDITH SHAMIAN

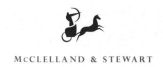

McCLELLAND & STEWART

Library and Archives Canada Cataloguing in Publication

Shalof, Tilda, author
Bringing it home : a nurse discovers the world beyond the hospital / Tilda Shalof.

Issued in print and electronic formats.
ISBN 978-0-7710-8000-5 (pbk.).—ISBN 978-0-7710-8001-2 (html)

1. Nursing—Canada—Anecdotes. 2. Nursing—Social aspects—Canada—Anecdotes. 3. Nurses—Canada—Anecdotes. 4. Medical care—Canada—Anecdotes. 5. Shalof, Tilda. I. Title.

RT6.A1S53 2014   362.17'30971   C2013-906883-X
                                        C2013-906884-8

Published simultaneously in the United States of America by
McClelland & Stewart, a division of Random House of Canada Limited
P.O. Box 1030, Plattsburgh, New York 12901

Library of Congress Control Number: 2013938863

Cover design: Rachel Cooper
Cover image: © Emrah Turudu/Getty Images
Typeset by Erin Cooper
Printed and bound in the United States of America

McClelland & Stewart,
a division of Random House of Canada Limited,
A Penguin Random House Company
www.randomhouse.ca

1   2   3   4   5   18   17   16   15   14

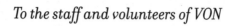

To the staff and volunteers of VON

CONTENTS

Foreword

by Judith Shamian

HOME IS A WORD THAT most associate with safety and security, a familiar place where we gather to be with the people we care about. It is therefore not surprising that most of us would prefer to be cared for at home if possible, and even die at home.

In spite of the fact it is so clear to all of us that getting well at home is more natural than in hospitals, the Canadian — as well as other countries' — health care system is built and judged by the availability of the acute care systems, meaning hospitals. Throughout the last two centuries, governments have consistently reinforced the message that having many hospitals, with the most up-to-date equipment, is the hallmark of good health care. But this does not reflect reality. There is no question that we need high-quality, sophisticated hospitals that can provide complex care to those who need it. But investing most of the health care dollars in the hospital sector (like many countries do) deprives the public of the care they need and deserve.

I came to Victorian Order of Nurses Canada in 2004 as its President and CEO after a rich working history in teaching hospitals, government, academia, and with some primary health care experience. With this background I was able to look at VON and quickly realize that it was a hidden jewel. It had been in existence for more than one hundred years, founded by Lady Aberdeen during Florence Nightingale's era to serve the underserved in their own community, in their own homes, based on their own needs. Today the buzz words in health care are "patient centered care." Many think that we in the 21st century discovered this revolutionary concept, yet it was already a defining part of VON's doctrine back in 1897. Over the years and against many odds, VON has made every effort to hang on to this notion. When I joined VON, I immediately became hooked on this philosophy and it became clear to me that so many countries still don't "get it." I felt that VON had a huge responsibility to educate the people and governments on why home, community care, and social services are essential to a healthy nation.

Fortunately, while I was formulating these thoughts around the essence of home, community, and social services, other organizations were also coming around to this thinking. These days most leading global agencies like the United Nations, World health Organization, World Bank, and many others advocate for "Universal Health Care Systems," where everyone, regardless of financial means, would have access to the care they need. While this sounds like a very reasonable goal, the truth is that it is rarely attained. One of the reasons that Universal Care is out of reach to many is because of the lack of home and community care systems. This major gap in our health care systems and profound lack of understanding of the importance of having integrated home and community services has driven me to take on the advocacy for the home and community care agenda.

To advocate, promote, fight, and influence can be done in many ways. This wonderful book by Tilda Shalof is one of the means by which we can advance the home and community care programs. Many people, including nurses themselves, do not even know what home care is until they need it — and then they see how poor the system is. One of the myths we need to dispel is that home care is just about visiting the elderly. By reading these stories you will get a glimpse of the variety and great value of home care. As Tilda and I discuss early in the book, most health care professionals do not value and do not understand the role of those who work in the home and the community care sector. This book showcases those highly skilled, hard-working individuals. As a proud nurse as well as a health care executive, I believe it is important that we understand the role and the contribution that these silent heroes play. Without volunteers, family members, personal support workers, in addition to nurses and others, we could not provide the support and care people deserve in their own home.

From an economic perspective, it is important to understand that home, community, and social services are the most cost-effective and impactful solutions. Canada spends less than five percent of our health care dollars on this sector – which is a serious flaw in our health care system. Many other countries spend three to four times more than Canada does and the relationship is clear: countries that have better home, community, and social services have better over-all health status.

As you will read in these pages, I had a difficult time convincing Tilda to write this book. I could have asked various authors but I was set on Tilda. Tilda is the "Nurse Cherry Ames" of the 21st Century, to reference a heroic (but fictional) character. Her previous books showed me that she is the kind of nurse that we want to see working in this profession all over the world. Tilda is a smart, caring, engaged, and personable nurse. She advocates for her patients and families while working collaboratively with the rest of the health care team, which can be a fine line to tread. She has an ability to capture the reality of the nursing world and to make us feel part of the story. So I knew I needed her to say yes to this important and challenging project – to tell the real story of nursing care in the home and the community.

I want to thank Tilda for saying "YES" and going on this journey with the most amazing staff, families, and clients. For eight years I was privileged to be at the helm of this incredible organization and I am extremely proud of the valuable work VON has been doing in Canada for over 110 years. My hope is that when you read *Bringing It Home*, you will share in the experiences of those giving and receiving this care, and ultimately understand why we must support these programs.

1

NAYSAYING

"NO!"

"No way."

"Big mistake, Tilda. Don't do it."

Then the kicker: "You'll never come back. No one does."

That's my fear, too. There's something about the hospital that makes a nurse think, *If I leave, I'll never go back.*

Our nursing station chatter ends with the approach of a stretcher, the high-pitched beeps of a cardiac monitor becoming increasingly louder. My patient has arrived from the operating room, swarmed by a bevy of serious people in green scrubs: the surgeon and her residents, an anesthesiologist, an OR nurse, a respiratory technologist, and a porter. A fresh liver transplant. Six IV pumps, a unit of blood hanging, oxygen set at 100 per cent. I eyeball the cardiac monitor – heart rate 136, sinus tachycardia, blood pressure 82 over 44. Oxygen sats 85 per cent. No urine in the urometer. Diagnosis: a sick patient and a busy night ahead for me.

The surgeons go into a huddle. I listen to a verbal report from the OR nurse and the anesthesiologist while the rest of the team attends to the patient. Ashley attaches cardiac electrodes to his chest so that

Belle can connect the cables to the monitors. Riccardo orders a stat chest x-ray, draws arterial blood gases and a slew of other blood tests. Charity calibrates transducers, zeroes pumps, and records starting totals of each infusion. Edna hangs a bag of blood. Jasna sees the mean arterial pressure has dropped to 59 mm Hg so she titrates the Levophed drip up from 0.021 mcg per kg per minute to 0.030. The patient's oxygen saturations are only 84 per cent on 100 per cent oxygen, so Manju, the respiratory therapist, increases the FiO_2. I'm ready to approach my patient, introduce myself, and begin my head-to-toe assessment, starting with "head"; my patient is deeply sedated, unconscious, and unresponsive.

What could beat this – the excitement of a new admission? Working together to save someone's life? It's energizing, even exhilarating – why would I ever leave? How could I be a nurse without a crisis, without everything at stake?

We work steadily into the night. The distraught wife and son stand on either side of the bed holding their loved one's hand. They try to read our faces and decipher the machines and monitors. As I go about caring for her husband, his father, I answer their questions and explain every single thing I do. They can see the situation is serious, getting worse, and I don't deny it. An abdominal ultrasound proves what we suspect: internal bleeding.

"Your husband is not doing well," the surgeon says. "He has to go back to the OR."

The mother and son are shocked. We prepare the patient to return to the operating room. I put my arm around her. This is good news, I tell them. We can fix this problem.

In the ICU, there are occasional ebbs in the frenetic flow, little lulls when you can take a break and tune out, even rest and think. One of those times is when your patient goes to the OR. First, I check the arrest cart to make sure it's well stocked, and then I ask around if anyone needs help. Tonight I'm on a mission. I'm conducting a survey.

As I make my way around the ICU with a clipboard on my hip, I stop at every room to ask each nurse a question.

"Home care. What's your first thought?"

In research, n refers to the number of subjects, and my n is nine. Here are the findings:

"I don't know anything about home care. Isn't it just chit-chatting with people?"

"Is home care the same as public health?"

"Sound's boring. A snoozefest. I'd lose my ICU skills."

"It's too slow, too much paperwork. You're out there on your own. No team."

"It doesn't pay as much as the hospital."

"You have to go into creepy homes. It's dangerous and I'm not prepared to put myself at risk."

"My uncle was rude to his home care nurse and she just took it. I didn't like that."

"It's just clipping old ladies' toenails and getting people to their doctor's appointments, isn't it?"

Only Riccardo has something positive to say. "Home care nurses made it possible for my grandmother to be at home in her last years and die there. Why not care for people in their homes where they want to be rather than in the hospital where no one wants to be?"

I slip into the Wellness Room, provided for us by Denise, our manager. It's a quiet place to read, watch TV, or lie down. I sit on the recliner and put my feet up to mull things over. I have a decision to make.

Before coming to work, I spent the afternoon with a prominent leader of the nursing profession, Dr. Judith Shamian. We'd met a few times before on the nursing conference circuit, where I entertain audiences with stand-up comedy nurse jokes and my funny/sad, heartwarming/heart-wrenching ICU stories, and where Judith lectures on nursing leadership, health care policy, global health, and, generally, how to make the world a better place. In my world, Judith is a big deal, a "who's who" – the closest we have to a celebrity. Out of the blue, she called me up and invited me to stop by her house for a visit. I assumed it was purely social, as she'd explained that Saturday is her only day for visiting with people. She is über-busy and is out of town a lot. She has more titles than a library – president of this, professor of that, and, currently, CEO of the Victorian Order of Nurses, "a homecare and community support organization," according to a VON brochure she gave me to read.

For some time, I have wondered why someone as brilliant and highly educated, as dynamic and visionary as Judith Shamian would be involved with something as old-fashioned and dreary – as Mickey Mouse and rinky-dink – as home care nursing. And as for the Victorian Order of Nurses? That dinosaur is history, a part of Canadian folklore, a horse-and-buggy operation, with pioneer roots dating back to the Klondike Gold Rush and Spanish influenza outbreak.

When I arrived at her modest, midtown home, Judith met me at the door before I even had a chance to ring the bell, and I suddenly realized why. Judith is Jewish – I am, too, but she's an *Orthodox* Jew and would not want the electric doorbell to be rung on a Saturday, the Jewish Sabbath. She wore a plain navy dress, dark stockings, and low-heeled patent pumps, which seemed like formal attire for a day of rest at home. I felt a bit out of place, casually dressed in jeans and a purple sweatshirt with a big pink tie-dyed heart. My scrubs were packed in my knapsack for changing into in the hospital locker room.

Judith and I greeted one another warmly, exchanging pleasantries and compliments about each other's recent, albeit minuscule, weight loss. She offered tea or coffee and I followed her into her large kitchen. On the counter there was a pair of tall silver candlesticks with hardened wax dripping down the sides. They had been lit the evening before, Friday at sundown, to welcome the Sabbath.

Judith drew hot water from a preheated urn. I was going to request tea, which I take black, but decided to ask for coffee, which I take with milk, so that she would open her refrigerator. A quick glance confirmed what I suspected: it was dark inside. Before sundown on Friday, she'd disconnected the light bulb so that electricity wouldn't be activated by opening the door. (It is permissible to avail oneself of electricity but not to activate or deactivate it.)

From the kitchen we moved out to her elegant, simply furnished living room. It had an old-world, European feeling, with elegant furniture and heavy oil paintings on the wall hanging next to framed children's drawings. We settled in front of a large bay window, into two comfortable chairs, turned slightly toward each other. A small antique table between us was piled with books and journals. A quick peek at their spines revealed eclectic interests – a copy of *The Economist*, a detective novel, a book called *To Heal a Fractured World*, and a well-worn Hebrew prayer book. I'm sure that on every other day of the week Judith reads electronically, but not on the Sabbath.

I had brought her a copy of my latest book as a gift and she seemed delighted to receive it. However, when I reached into my knapsack for a pen to write an inscription, she held up her hand and placed it lightly on my arm. "Would you please sign it for me another time?"

Of course. In this house, writing is forbidden on the Sabbath.

Orthodox Jews mystify me. In addition to the famous "Top Ten" commandments, they follow an additional 613 laws that rabbis and other scholars have identified from the bible.

As for me, I unreliably observe maybe three or four – give or take, hit or miss – and only the fun ones involving foods and presents, not the uncomfortable or inconvenient ones involving restrictions and prohibitions. As for observing the Sabbath the way Judith does, I can't fathom the idea of disconnecting from the world for even an hour, much less an entire day every week, not to mention the numerous holidays and festivals around the year, each requiring abstinence from work and adherence to rules and prohibitions.

Judith and I are professional *acquaintances*. We aren't friends, though I'd like to be. She's not my mentor, though I wish she were.

She's warm and friendly, but *formidable* and slightly intimidating, though I don't think she means to be. Her intelligence is fierce and her energy legendary. She is a force to be reckoned with. The age difference between us is only about ten years, but we move in different circles and she's way out of my league. Yet, we do share important things in common – our belief that the sun rises and sets with nursing, and that nursing is the solution to most of the world's problems.

With her impressive academic credentials, scientific chops, and political savvy, Judith is working toward that vision. Bedside nursing, management, research, teaching, policy development, multiple university degrees (earned and honorary), awards, papers published – she's done many things. My career has been dedicated to one: working in the intensive care unit and writing about it. (That's two things, but who's counting?)

I asked her, "What's your secret to accomplishing so much?"

She smiled serenely. "The Sabbath. It recharges me."

So, a day of rest makes her *more* productive, not less. Interesting.

"But how did you manage to do it all – a master's degree, then a Ph.D., have a high-powered career, manage a home, raise a family of three, and be a grandmother to sixteen?"

"I'm not going to tell you it's easy. It's not. The juggling is constant. But if you have a true partner, it's possible."

I wondered where her husband was. "He's still at *shul*," she said. "*Shabbes* is almost over." She used the old-school, Yiddish terms for synagogue and Sabbath.

Then she asked me something that took me by surprise. "How would you like to write a book about home care and VON?"

"No, thank you," I answered politely. "I don't know much about home care."

That was a lie. I know *nothing* about home care. I write about what I know, what I'm passionate about. Like a lot of people, Judith must think I can cobble together a book out of thin air, whip one up, easy-peasy. (It's like the joke about the neurosurgeon and the author. They're at a party and the neurosurgeon says to the author that he'd like to write a book, so the author says he'd like to do some neurosurgery.)

"You could learn about home care," Judith says, responding to my objection. "What if I were to send you on a trip across the country to visit VON sites, see our programs in action, meet staff, volunteers, and, most of all, our clients?"

Clients. Oh, sure. They taught us that term in nursing school. It's an attempt to give the impression we're all on equal footing, but no one believes that and no one ever actually uses the term *client*, certainly not in the hospital. And, take it from me, I've been on the other side, the receiving end of hospital care, and when you are lying in that bed, you are a *patient*.

"Isn't home care driving around, checking up on people in their homes?"

"What VON does is much more than that." Briefly, she looked at me askance, like *Maybe I'm wrong about you.* "Yes, home care is caring for people in their homes, but it's also about preventing illness, teaching people about their health and how to manage chronic diseases, and much more. It's about primary care and helping people stay independent and keeping them out of institutions. It's for all ages and takes place in a house, or a community centre, school, church, even on a street corner or in a back alley crack house. It involves nurses, doctors, volunteers, family caregivers, home care workers, case managers, social workers, nurse practitioners, and others."

I looked at the brochure she'd given me. "VON – Health Starts at Home." Doesn't health start and end in the hospital? That's how it's always seemed to me.

We sat quietly. I looked at my watch and drained my coffee cup. I had to get going soon. Night shift starts precisely at 1915 hours and it's frowned upon to be late, as well as inconsiderate to the tired day shift nurse who's waiting to give the handover report and go home. But as I got up to leave, Judith asked me another question. This one took me aback even more than her first. It surprised, but then rankled, me.

"Why aren't there more nurse leaders? Why aren't more nurses involved in the bigger issues of our profession, like policy development or health care reform? Why don't nurses speak up about important issues, or engage in social activism or political advocacy?"

Easy for you to say. When's the last time you worked a night shift or a long weekend? When's the last time you changed a dressing, gave a bed bath, or ran to a Code Blue? You're just another out-of-touch academic in your ivory tower. How disappointing!

I must have looked as perplexed as I felt, because she explained further.

"Yes, there are nurses on Parliament Hill lobbying to implement policy changes and one or two running as political candidates. Others speak out against homelessness and poverty. There are nurses who work in clinics for refugees who have no health care coverage. These are wonderful contributions, but why are they so few in number and the rest remain silent? We now have the most educated cohort of nurses in history, yet so few are in corporate management or global leadership. Nurses will continue to be left behind."

I felt myself getting annoyed with her grandiose questions. "What nurse has the time or the energy for any of that? Do you have any idea of a nurse's workload? The responsibilities? Patient care takes everything out of us. Why isn't it enough to be a front-line nurse, giving patient care?" Her questions irked me. I was steamed up and let it rip. "Most of us are already stretched to the limit between shift work, caring for our patients, and our families at home. Do you have any idea how many nurses are also caring for a family member at home? Are we supposed to take care of the world? Why don't academics like you, with all of your university degrees, know anything about real, hands-on nursing?" I picked up my knapsack from the floor. *If I leave now, I'll make it to work on time.*

"There are three kinds of nurses," Judith said evenly, continuing with her lecture, taking no notice of my ruffled feathers. "The first type of nurse takes care of patients. For this nurse, patient care is enough. The second type of nurse is a researcher or an educator, but disconnected from front-line realities. This nurse may be involved in charitable causes or political activism, but separates that work from their identity as a nurse. They get nursing amnesia and forget that they are nurses."

"I'm the first type," I snapped. "I like taking care of patients. It's why I went into nursing and why I stay." I walked to the door before she could expound on the third type.

Judith accompanied me to the door. "I'm leaving for Geneva, Switzerland, tomorrow for a meeting at the World Health Organization. In two weeks when I get back, VON will be holding our annual general meeting in Windsor, Ontario. Perhaps you could join us at the AGM, where you can meet some of the key people at VON."

And who might they be? Florence Nightingale, the Lady with the Lamp? Clara Barton of the Red Cross? Maybe the ghost of Lady Ishbel Aberdeen, founder of VON in 1897, according to the brochure which I'd already crumpled into my knapsack and planned to toss out when I got to work.

"Think it over," she continued, now smiling, our heated debate forgotten. "Wait until after you experience the AGM to decide your answer."

"I'll let you know," I said and turned away. I already knew my answer.

I stepped out onto the porch. The sky was dark and three stars twinkled above. The Sabbath was over. A trim, handsome man in a suit carrying a folded white-and-blue-striped prayer shawl in a clear bag – it must be Judith's husband – was coming up the stairs, arriving home. "Have a good week," he said to me.

As I drove to work, all I could think of was how to brush off Judith's offer. *Maybe she'll drop it after that testy exchange? Surely she sees how far apart we are?* She must have sensed my lukewarm reaction to her proposal. How could I even think about leaving the hospital, even temporarily? It's what I know best. It's my *home*.

For the past thirty years, I have been a hospital nurse, most of that time in this same Medical-Surgical Intensive Care Unit of the Toronto General Hospital. I've worked hard to master the ICU, acquire the skills, stay on top of my game, and keep my edge. Over the years, I'd dabbled in a few other things – floor nursing and a few shifts in the emergency department. I'd made a half-hearted attempt at graduate school to do a master's degree in nursing, but I dropped out after the first semester. Oh, and nine summers of camp nursing – that was a fun adventure. But after each bold foray away from the ICU, I returned to my comfort zone. Let's face it: I'm a lifer, addicted to the rush, the human dramas, the controlled chaos, even the noise, mess, and pace. I love supporting families through a crisis. I thrive on the danger of septic shock, the ooziness of end-stage liver disease, the complexity of rare autoimmune disorders – not to mention "everyday" respiratory failure and lethal cardiac arrhythmias. Even after all these years, I still find critical care fascinating. Where I work, we are doing fascinating research and implementing cutting-edge technology, such as incubating stem cells and growing new organs in the laboratory. We are caring for patients on extracorporeal life support (ECLS) to oxygenate blood and remove carbon dioxide outside of a person's body.

My break is over. Time to get back to work. I leave the calm of the Wellness Room and re-enter the fray. Tamara's patient is a young woman on an artificial lung device that will hopefully bridge her over until she might receive a life-saving transplant. Kate is caring for an elderly man in acute respiratory distress syndrome who's on the high-speed oscillating ventilator and may have to be placed on ECLS. I see Jasna titrating down the inotropes her patient is on for low blood pressure, so he must be improving. Janet, who's on the mobile ICU dream team, and had been roaming the floors, scouting for patients in distress, is now rushing into the ICU with a patient who's gone into florid pulmonary edema and needs intubation, *stat*. (I better get in there and help her.)

At 0520 hours my patient returns from the OR to the ICU, this time with a smaller and more relaxed caravan in tow. The surgery went well. His blood pressure is 118 over 78, normal sinus rhythm at 72 per minute. Only two IV infusions running now. Urine is flowing. It's time

to empty drains, zero pumps, tally up ins and outs, finish my charting, and organize my thoughts in order to give a coherent report to
the day nurse.

What could be better than this? More rewarding? More *exciting*?
When Judith gets back in town, I'll call her to tell her my unequivocal
answer: No.

2

FIFTY SHADES OF NURSING

IN THE MORNING after last night's shift, before driving home and toddling off to bed, I attend a meeting of the Bagel Club. There are four of us today: me (aka Tillie), Janet (aka "the Grand Pooh-Bah"), Jasna (aka "Jazzy"), and Stephanie ("Shorty"). As we sit reviewing the night, eating (bagels, what else?), and knitting colourful socks (Janet calls it "sockology"), I tell them about Judith's offer of cross-country travel and a writing assignment.

"You're not seriously thinking of doing it, are you?" Janet looks at me dubiously. Two more pairs of dubious eyes look at me over their knitting needles.

"Maybe. I'm not sure." I prevaricate, not even sure why I am now wavering. Last night, I was so certain. Aside from Judith's proposal, I wanted to talk with them about the questions she'd asked me just before I left. I looked around the circular table at my friends. They are all outstanding nurses who also do the yeoman's share of care-giving in their families – one for a profoundly developmentally delayed son who requires twenty-four-hours-a-day supervision, another as a single mother raising teenagers on her own, and so on. In addition to full-time hospital work and at-home responsibilities, they're each involved in volunteering and fundraising for causes such as cancer research and autism treatment. I think of others I know, like Muriel, who also works full-time and cares for her aged father-in-law, who lives in their home. There's Omar, who has put his travel plans on hold to stay and care for his vibrant but frail ninety-year-old mother. Wendy's father just had major surgery and she's taken time off work to care for him. And others. Most of us have someone we're worried about.

As soon as I get home, I dash off an email.

Dear Judith,

Thank you for our visit. I've been thinking over the question you raised about why more front-line nurses don't get involved in professional issues, policy development, politics, etc. Frankly, I am amazed at those who do, given the demands of a nursing career. There's a huge separation between the practitioners of our profession and nursing scholars. Perhaps more academics need to learn about front-line nursing. After all, isn't research supposed to be about improving patient care?? Doesn't it start there? I invite you to a meeting of the Bagel Club to learn about the reality of working nurses' lives and concerns.

I press Send. Within minutes I receive a reply.

Wow. This is the BEST email I've had in ages. Your reflections help me understand so much. Right now, I am flying to Thunder Bay to visit health clinics in First Nations reserves, then back to the University of Toronto. Later in the week, I'll be in Ottawa, meeting the minister of health and your words will be foremost in my mind. Thank you for the invitation to your group. Judith.

I write back: *Do you knit?*

I have a talent – some call it a gift – for sleeping. After a few hours of slumber, I awake in the afternoon like a bear emerging from hibernation, refreshed and ready for spring. After rest and reconsideration, last night's adamant *no* has morphed into a tentative *maybe*. But it's not just sleep that's brought about my change of heart; it has something to do with catching sight of Dr. Margaret Herridge this morning after last night's shift. Just as I was stumbling bleary-eyed out of the hospital, I saw her striding briskly in, coffee cup in hand, energetic and eager to get at her day. We waved, but didn't stop to chat as we usually do. (No energy for me, no time for her.) Margaret is one of the medical directors of our ICU, a world-renowned researcher and a wise and caring doctor. Seeing Margaret reminded me that for the past ten years, she's been studying the aftermath of critical illness. She follows former ICU patients, visiting them at home to learn about their recovery.

When I arrived home, just before going to bed, I turned on the computer to watch a YouTube video of Margaret discussing her research findings. She's wearing a white lab coat over an elegant suit. There's her classically beautiful face looking genuinely concerned as she speaks to the camera.

"We previously assumed that ICU survivors got back to normal and returned to their regular lives. However, that is not the case." Margaret goes on to describe the ongoing physical and psychological problems of ICU survivors and the enormous burden of caregiving shouldered by overextended, exhausted family members.

Yes, I'd also always assumed it was happily-ever-after for our patients at home. But now that I think of it, even one of our most famous lung transplant patients, Hélène Campbell (whose organ donor awareness campaign gained the support of Justin Bieber and Ellen DeGeneres), took more than a year to recover at home, and still has ongoing health issues.

"Five years after surviving a critical illness, many patients remain physically fragile and suffer post-traumatic stress disorder [PTSD] from an ICU stay," Margaret reports on the video.

When I ask her about it a few days later after team rounds, during a day shift in the ICU, she tells me more. "It's a growing public health issue. We invest so much in critically ill patients in the hospital, but almost nothing when they're at home recovering." She suggests I visit a few of our past ICU patients to see for myself.

Richard immediately springs to mind. I don't usually stay in touch with patients (some nurses develop ongoing friendships, including visits, Facebook, et cetera), but Richard-Thornton Sharp and his husband, Jim Harris, were an exception for many of us. They were such a warm and loving couple, and their kindness extended to the entire staff. They got to know us as individuals, and the affectionate feelings were mutual. For the first few weeks after Richard went home, a few of the ICU nurses and respiratory therapists took turns staying overnight to ease the transition. Unfortunately, he has had to be readmitted to the ICU a few times due to recurring lung infections.

In their east-end townhouse, I sit with Richard in his book-, art-, and music-filled office. Jim is at work but will be home soon. Richard reminds me how his medical problem started. He developed a thymus gland tumour that crept into his chest, encroached into his lungs, and threatened to obstruct his airway.

"One day I passed out in the grocery store." He pauses to breathe. "I fell on top of a cheese display. Fortunately, it broke my fall." He indraws a quick breath.

"At least it was soft." I finish the joke for him because he doesn't have the energy to do so himself. He nods in thanks.

Then came surgery, multiple complications, and a year-long ICU stay filled with gradual, tedious progress and frequent drastic setbacks. There were even periods of time when Richard was awake and walking, but still critically ill. (How is that possible, you ask? Trust me. We see it all the time.) A tall, majestically handsome man who was once a Shakespearean actor, Richard is now frail and weak, but still nicely dressed in a crisp blue-striped shirt and casual pants. His hands tremble and his voice wavers as he pours me a cup of tea.

"Wearing clothes marked a return from my patient costume back to my civilian uniform, but I hardly have the strength to button my shirts. In the hospital, I worked so hard with Vince, the ICU physiotherapist who knew just how to motivate me. Vince gave me the confidence that I could get better, even run a hundred miles. I've lost all of that now."

Jim arrives home and greets me with a bear hug, just like the ones he gave all of us during his daily visits to Richard in the ICU. I try to hide my shock at Jim's haggard appearance. Once robust and jovial, Jim is now a shadow of his former self, gaunt and tense-looking. He rakes his hand through his hair in frustration. "I love Richard, but it's going to ruin our marriage if I have to be his full-time caregiver. We get a few hours a week of home care, but I'm on duty all the rest of the time and every night."

Richard nods in agreement. "Family and friends have pitched in to help Jim. Respiratory therapists and nurses from the hospital have spelled him off. We had everything we needed in the hospital and nothing here at home. The assumption was always that Jim would be my full-time caregiver."

"I felt bullied into it," Jim admits. "I had no choice. Yes, I wanted Richard home, but I was terrified and completely overwhelmed. Suddenly, I had to be the RN, MD, PT, and RT. I had to manage his pills, ventilator, tracheostomy care, plus shopping, cooking, and also hold down my job to support us. We have put together a team of helpful people, but we can't sustain it. Everyone has lives of their own."

The burden of caregiving. If only love were enough. . . . How well I know.

"All of our dreams – gone," Jim says. "Retirement, growing old together, travel – kaput. I'm on no sleep, constantly listening for alarms, getting up during the night to troubleshoot the ventilator. Then I go to work in the morning. The hospital saves your life but then throws you under the bus. Sometimes I want to say, take him back, I can't handle it."

I'm surprised he says this in front of Richard, but Richard nods sympathetically to Jim about the burdens that caring for him has imposed.

"When I came home I was like a corpse," Richard says over the low hiss of the oxygen tank. "Jim had to do everything for me. I could barely walk to the bathroom. I could hardly speak. To have a shower was my daily Everest."

"The support I have for Richard is wonderful, but I need more," Jim says. "The ICU team worked so hard with him. How can we let that slide now at home?"

I leave wondering when, and if, I will see them again. Richard's condition is terminal. Their difficult situation weighs heavily on my mind. I like problems, but only ones I can solve. Sometimes it feels like there's never enough nursing care.

Dr. Herridge had filled me in about the progress of another of our ICU patients, whom I also remember well. Pat and her husband, Ken Hillcoff, are home now, after a lengthy ICU stay. Pat developed end-stage kidney disease and is dependent on frequent hemodialysis, which they now do at home. Hemodialysis is a major procedure for any patient, involving heavy machines, technical skills, expertise, and sound clinical judgement. I can't believe it's possible to do it at home for any patient, much less Pat, whose condition can become unstable quickly. This I have to see. What's next? Outpatient cardiac surgery? Drive-by appendectomies?

When I call Pat and Ken, they remember me well and invite me over for a visit at their high-rise condo. When Pat opens the door I gasp. She is drop-dead gorgeous – glamorous, even. Out on the street, I wouldn't have even recognized her, though once, I knew every part of her body, inside and out. Dressed in a black sparkly blouse, black trousers, and sporting bright red nails, she looks ready for a night at the opera. Next, it startled me to hear her voice – so much of a person's identity, but something I'd never heard, even though I'd conversed with Pat for almost a year. (We rarely get to hear our patients' voices because most are unconscious and almost all are intubated and on ventilators.)

"I am reluctant to tell my story," Pat starts slowly. "It's scary for people to hear."

"Yes, but look at you now. You're a success story. That gives people hope."

Her husband, Ken, is the same attentive, easygoing gentleman I got to know in the ICU. He visited Pat every day and sat for hours at her bedside. "I'm semi-retired now," he says, "which is good because I have the time to look after Pat."

"Ken looks at life positively, so I have no choice but to be positive, too," Pat says.

"My husband is like that, too," I say. "Brutal, isn't it?" We commiserate about our eternally optimistic husbands.

Like Richard, Pat flip-flopped between being terribly ill and being extremely ill. She had a fatal lung disease and received a double lung transplant, but then got every possible complication – infections, bleeding, blood clots, kidney failure, and organ rejection. I was Pat's nurse when she first came back from the OR. Her surgery was so deep and extensive that the surgeons couldn't close her huge incision. For weeks she stayed in a medically induced coma with her chest open. We could peer inside and watch her heart beat and her lungs rise and fall.

"You were on ECMO. Do you remember?" What *does* she remember of her lengthy, arduous ICU ordeal?

"Ken told me a lot but I don't remember much. Thankfully," she adds with a shudder.

Pat now knows all about the extracorporeal membrane osmosis machine that took over her lung functions for a few weeks. She was in the hospital for three hundred days and has ongoing medical problems such as kidney failure, requiring frequent hemodialysis.

"One day, as I was walking through the hospital, I saw an office with a sign on the door," Ken recounts. "It said 'Home Dialysis.' I assumed it meant a nurse would come to our house to do it for us, but they told me we would do it ourselves. 'An ordinary civilian can do this? How is that possible?' That was my first thought."

"My first thought was how scared I was," Pat says, her voice trembling.

Ken reaches over to stroke her hand. "At first, they didn't think Pat would be a suitable candidate because her condition is complicated. She is very sensitive to fluid shifts. If I take off the blood too quickly her blood pressure drops, but then I decrease the rate of ultra-filtration or give her a saline bolus. I've learned to draw up the heparin syringe, set up the machine, prime the tubing and the filter. I know how to detect blood clots or air bubbles that can get in there. If her blood coagulates and I can't return it to her, her hemoglobin drops and she gets weak. Then we have to go to the hospital for a transfusion. I knew how unstable she is, but still, we wanted to give it a try. It would give us independence, not to mention the convenience. So, we took classes four days a week. I had watched Nurse Celine for months and felt that with her help I could master it. Now, it's great. We go at our speed and do it when it suits us. Now, Pat can drink as much as she wants, and if her weight is up because she's retaining fluids, and her lungs get wet and she gets short of breath, we just do an extra run. Pat's condition can change fast, as you know, so I monitor her closely. What works best for Pat is to do three days in a row, then one day off."

"Sometimes I feel fluid rushing to my lungs, so I have oxygen, if I need it," Pat says.

"A lot of it is emotional," Ken explains. "I know how to calm Pat down. We do our mindfulness breathing techniques that Dr. Susan Abbey taught us. Nurse Celine came to our home many times. She'd be sneaky, creeping up to set off an alarm or clamp off tubing, just to see what I would do. Celine gave me her home number and said I could call anytime. I've never used it, but it's reassuring to have it."

"Tell Tilda about the scary thing that happened," Pat prompts.

"One day there was a snow storm and the power went off. The machine only has a ten-minute battery and we were in the middle of dialysis."

"I panicked," Pat says. "I took an Ativan to calm me down. We had to stop dialysis, and my blood clotted in the filter and couldn't be returned to me. But that's the worst thing that's happened."

In a few hours, the power came back on and they were able to proceed with dialysis.

Ken explains more. "Before we took this on, a hospital technologist came to check if there was enough space, power, and adequate water pressure. The hospital supplies everything. All we have to pay is the increased cost of electricity and water. It's the equivalent of water running for six hours per treatment. Then, of course, there's my nursing wages. Fortunately, they're zero." Ken shoots first Pat, then me, a wink. "It's cost-effective for the hospital, not to mention the benefits to our quality of life. But it's not for everyone."

Pat's chief complaint now is a disturbing one: frequent nightmares and terrifying ICU flashbacks. "I'm right back there. IV poles are swaying from the ceiling and metal panels are swinging at me as I try to dodge them like in a car wash." She shudders. "I have flashbacks to one particular night when I had a blood clot in my lungs. Do you remember that, Tilda?"

"I'll be honest with you, Pat. You had so many crises, I can't remember them all."

"Once, in the middle of the night, they had to take me for a CT scan. This hunched old man was pushing me along a dimly lit hallway. The hospital was eerie, quiet, and dark. The radiologist read me the list of all the things that could go wrong. 'Death' was on that list. This has all the makings for a horror movie, I thought. It was very surreal."

"What helps you deal with your PTSD?" I ask.

"Dr. Abbey, the psychiatrist at the hospital, taught me how to meditate and do mindfulness practice. She did it with me in her office. That meant a lot to me. What a trust it sets up between patient and doctor. She didn't say, 'Go home and do this yourself.' We did it together. Now, I do it during dialysis or whenever I become anxious."

"Pat has a way of working herself up into a state," Ken says in a soothing voice.

It's time to set up the machine and begin Pat's dialysis. "Stringing the machine is the easy part," Ken explains, confidently winding plastic tubing through levers, spools, and valves, and priming the filter.

"Ken dear, let's change me into an open-necked top so you can get to my dialysis port more easily." Tenderly, Ken removes Pat's sparkly blouse, undoes her bra, and slips a loose T-shirt over her head. On the shirt it says, "Don't take your organs to heaven. Heaven knows we need them here." Ken touches her body like he's handling a treasure, though not necessarily a fragile one. "We work together," he says. "I keep my mind on the machine and Pat reminds me if I forget anything."

"You two make dialysis romantic." While they set up the machine, I leave them alone for a few minutes and look around their apartment. There are beautiful things on display, lots of books on walnut shelves; nothing is out of place, nothing superfluous, no clutter.

When I come back Pat tells me, "I now like beer and football. That's new for me. Do you think I got that from my donor? But even before my lung transplant, I was complicated and sensitive and that hasn't changed." Pat remembers something else. "Do you remember you gave me a manicure one night? It meant so much to me."

I wonder if she remembers what else I did. She does.

"You asked if you could use my polish," Pat says. "You put 'Va-va-va-voom Red' on your nails so that we matched."

Guilty as charged.

"I also remember one night eavesdropping on your telephone conversation when you called home to speak to your children. It was one of your sons, after his hockey game."

"That sounds like me."

Pat has more ICU recollections. "I remember Dr. Herridge's kindness. Oh, and Dr. Lazar apologizing to me for being so blunt, but I told him I wanted to hear the truth. One day, in my foggy stupor, I heard a nurse say, 'She's never going to make it out of here.' I'm sure she didn't know I heard. That was hard to hear. I was very down after that."

We tend to assume our patients can't hear us; we'd better think again.

The machine whirls away and Pat and Ken manage confidently. I marvel at the courage it takes to do this.

"Nurse Celine calls to check on us from time to time, but at home, you're the doctor, technologist, nurse, inventory clerk, order desk, and physiotherapist," Ken says with obvious pride at what they've accomplished together.

Suddenly, I have my own ICU flashback – to Mr. Kadourian. He had end-stage renal disease just like Pat and was on home dialysis, competently managed by his wife, Zenia. But when Mr. K was admitted to the ICU with respiratory problems, we took over his dialysis and basically shut her out. Once, Zenia went over to change the dialysate bags because they were empty. A nurse rushed in to stop her and told her, not as nicely as she could have, "Don't interfere with our work. Here, we're in control." Yet, Zenia had been managing his care, running his dialysis at home, for years. She knew more about how to run a dialysis machine than we did and, of course, she knew everything about her husband. Like most family caregivers, she'd become an expert on his medical condition.

Pat's memories evoke more memories. "The ventilator. First I hated it, then I loved it. As for pain, yes, there were times when I had pain, but I was never left in pain." She glances at the dialysis machine. "Arterial pressures are high today, Ken dear." He gets up to tinker with the settings. "There's always something, but Ken will sort it out."

"Do you have any good memories of the ICU?"

"My best memory is Vince, the physiotherapist. Whenever I would say, 'I don't think I can do this, but I'll try,' Vince would say to me in Yoda's voice, 'Do or do not. There is no try.' He even brought me a little green Yoda action figure that talks. It was Vince who got me walking again."

Both Richard and Pat had mentioned Vince. I once asked him how he motivates patients. "Recovery is hard work. It's boot camp," he said. "Most of us would rather stay in bed than face that. The trick is to remind them of home. Focusing on going home makes patients push through the pain. Home is the biggest incentive, isn't it?"

Yes, *home* – it's what everyone wants.

Ken shows me his spreadsheets. There's one for recording Pat's medications, another for vital signs, and another for inventory and ordering supplies. "I've got it all under control."

He certainly does. They both do.

Wendy is a nurse who's always got her "Zen" on. She's utterly unflappable, calm and steady, logical and clear-thinking, no matter what emergency comes up. "Nothing stresses me," she admits, "except when my father got sick." She's invited me over to meet her father and mother, John and Mary Hunter, in the cozy suburban bungalow where Wendy grew up.

"Devastating."

Straightaway, that's what John says when I ask how his surgery went. He's a tall, handsome, tan gentleman, the picture of health despite his recent ordeal. In his white pressed shorts and white polo shirt, he looks ready for a tennis match. "A few months ago, I had bladder cancer, then surgery, radiation, and chemo. The surgeons left me with an 'ileal conduit,' which sounds a lot more glamorous than it really is," he says ruefully.

Taking his cue, I add, "Yes, it must be fun having surgery on your man parts and ending up with a urine bag attached to your abdomen."

"The hospital was horrific. The nurses would breeze in to ask, 'How's your pain?' How was my pain? It was like asking how long is a piece of string? Once I answered, 'Terrible,' and she went on a coffee break. The worst part was when I came home. Reality hit. They'd removed the tumour, but my bladder, ureters, prostate, lymph glands, were gone, too. I was a eunuch."

"It's like a hysterectomy," Wendy's mom, Mary, says. "They took away the baby carriage and left the playpen."

"*Fifty Shades of Grey* did nothing for me. That was another loss my libido. I remember when *Peyton Place* could get me going. *Tropic of Cancer*. Now, that's gone. But the most traumatic part was coming home with this bag and having no idea how to handle it."

I'm impressed how comfortable Wendy appears to be, listening to her father talk about his sex life. She looks at him so proudly and lovingly, grateful he is doing so well.

"Ursula was my home care nurse – make sure you use her real name in your book. She was beautiful, but when she handled me, I had no sensation. I received such cursory information in the hospital. I think I was in shock and didn't take it in. At first, when I got home, Wendy helped me. I couldn't face it. Then Ursula came to see me. I was entitled to eight visits, but near the end of my allotment, I still couldn't manage on my own. Ursula said, 'I'll keep coming until you don't need me.' She never gave up on me. One problem was the bag kept leaking. I couldn't get a seal. If the seal isn't perfect, acid gets on the skin and causes breakdown – you know this. I've since learned that there are many people walking around with bags like this. My heart cries for a young man with this thing." He pauses, thinking of something else. "Say, this book you're writing. Have you got a title for it?" In a flash, simultaneously, we both know a good one and say it in unison.

"Fifty Shades of Nursing!"

Yes, there are at least fifty. Maybe more.

3

PICTURES AT AN EXHIBITION

MY CURIOSITY IS PIQUED, which is why, a few weeks later, I find myself attending VON's annual general meeting. I still haven't given Judith my decision, but I'm keeping my options open. I've decided to decide after the AGM. It's being held this year in Windsor, Ontario, a small town on the U.S. border with Detroit, Michigan. Not an exotic locale, but with five hundred in attendance – mostly senior management, administrators, and board members – it requires the space of the huge ballroom of Caesars Hotel and Casino.

First thing I notice: they have a lot of meetings. I have an allergy to meetings; I break out in restlessness and impatience. In the hospital, our manager keeps our weekly staff meetings brisk and to the point. They're brief because we have to get back to work. For our patients and their families, the word *meeting* has a negative connotation. "Family meetings" always mean bad news. We never hold meetings to say the patient is improving, now, do we? One family used to beg us, "Please, no more meetings." They'd disappear whenever we tried to schedule one. That's how I'm beginning to feel; today's agenda is one meeting after another. During breaks, I mill around, hobnob with the crowd, drink coffee, and nibble on fruit and pastries. Feeling like an

interloper in foreign territory, I eavesdrop on their conversations and
try to figure out the unfamiliar jargon.

"CM for case manager is now CCC for care coordinator," someone
says. They frequently use the term "KT" and as I am puzzling over that,
they start speaking about "KPI."

I tap the person sitting next to me on the shoulder. "Psst. What's
KPI?"

"It's Key Performance Indicators," she whispers back and introduces
herself. Her name is Irene Holubiec, and she's a nurse who is the
senior director of quality and risk management. She helpfully inter-
prets these unfamiliar terms for me. But when they start talking about
"kaizen," and "lean," I am equally baffled. I'm just about to ask Irene
what these terms mean when one of the corporate suits gets up on the
podium to explain this management philosophy.

"Lean is flowing like a stream, no rocks or boulders disrupt the
flow. It's respect for the experts, those on the ground. It's about elim-
inating waste and non–value adding activity."

*Yeah, right. Come visit the hospital if you want to see disrupted flows,
obstacles, and waste.*

Between wandering in and out of meetings, and helping myself
to the snacks during the coffee breaks, I stroll around and manage to
pick up a few choice nuggets.

". . . the greatest expenditures in the health care system are in acute
care, yet hospital patients represent only 1 per cent of the population."

"Seniors now outnumber children. More of the population is over
sixty-five than under fifteen . . . this ratio is predicted to double as
baby boomers enter their sixties."

"Home care spending in Canada amounts to only 5 per cent of total
health care spending."

"Homelessness is a national disaster. Over thirty thousand
Canadians are homeless on any given day or night. . . . Poverty is the
single greatest risk factor for health."

"Health care to First Nations' communities like Sioux Lookout and

Attawapiskat is a disgrace . . . an 80 per cent rate of substance abuse and mental illness in this population."

"The future is about keeping people out of hospitals . . ."

"We drive people into institutions when support is not in place for them to stay home."

Yeah, yeah, yeah. These factoids could be lifted verbatim from my notes as a student nurse, circa 1983. Back then, they said the same things; nothing has changed. As for the vaunted "paradigm shift" that our instructors predicted – the movement away from the hospital to the community, the transition from an acute care, disease-focused health care system to a more preventive, primary care health care one – shows no signs of happening. To most people, *health care* means hospitals and doctors. We're still obsessed with medical interventions and the latest technology. In the huge, sprawling medical centre where I work, we offer "quaternary care"– above-and-beyond heroic measures for the most difficult cases. After primary care for prevention, secondary for early detection, and tertiary for acute problems, there's this fourth level of care. In fact, many of us who care for people with extraordinary and extreme medical conditions don't know much about basic first aid or even how to treat the common cold.

I leave the dark, cool casino and step out to the steaming pavement of a hot June afternoon to walk the streets of downtown Windsor. A down-and-out panhandler strums his guitar and chants his song: "No sex, no money, no love, no drugs. No sex, no money . . ." He stops, stoops down, picks up a cigarette butt, and attempts a few dry puffs. On either side of the street are out-of-business shops and boarded-up storefronts covered in graffiti. Pawn shops and a tattoo and piercing parlour: "Are You in Need of a New Hole?" There's a First Nations' detox clinic with dream catchers in the window, a new immigrant welcome centre. I walk back to the waterfront casino – with its ferris wheel, game arcade, and cotton candy – and return to the conference centre for more meetings. During a coffee break, I continue to

schmooze and mingle. I can feel the participants' passionate engagement. You'd be hard pressed to find so many positive attitudes in the
hospital. There, we go around looking grim and grumbling a lot. Here,
you'll hear things like:

"I feel motivated to support my staff to provide great care," a manager says.

"I love doing work that makes a real difference in people's lives,"
another enthuses.

"Where else do you get the opportunity to work and serve?"

VON seems to be one happy place. Yet, they are candid about the
problems in this venerable old institution. Their computer system is
outdated, their administration inefficient, and, worst of all, they've
lost market share and brand awareness. But they are working hard on
improvements. A senior member of the national board of directors, a
gentleman who looks like he's been around for awhile, provides the
background. "For years VON was a household name. You'd come home
from the hospital and a VON nurse would be there. Back then, hospital
stays were longer. Once, VON was synonymous with home care in
Canada," he says wistfully, "but not anymore."

"What happened?"

"It's a sad story." He looks very sad indeed. "Deregulation back in
the nineties led to competitive bidding and VON was ousted by big
businesses. A not-for-profit charity like VON couldn't compete with
big American corporations that moved in. Judith has worked to create
a hybrid of a business and charity model. She has streamlined our
administration and reorganized our operations. It used to take 227
steps from a referral to a nurse arriving at the client's doorstep. Now,
it's down to nine. We're determined to be the best once again."

Judith gets up on the podium to give the keynote address. She
opens with a quip about her version of CPR – Conviction. Passion.
Relationships. She says what everyone here already believes. "Home
care can no longer be an afterthought. It is the centre. Health care
must include home care for all. As Canadians, we value our universal

health care system and must protect and preserve it. There is absolutely no evidence that privatization of health care or for-profit health care benefits patients or saves money."

She speaks and everyone listens. No one is drifting off, no one is looking down at their phones. All eyes are on Judith. I notice she's pushed the microphone to the side so that the sound waves from her throat's vocal emanations will not be electronically transmitted on this Saturday afternoon. Even without amplification, Judith can easily project her resonant, Hungarian-accented voice, and considerable charisma, throughout the grand ballroom.

"Canada is world class in acute and critical care, but falls short in health promotion, disease prevention, and primary care. We have an illness care, not a health care, system."

She speaks about the need to empower the people on the ground, the ones actually providing care, by giving them the supports they need – technological, educational, et cetera – to care for clients. In particular, she praises the role of home care workers. "So often they feel invisible and undervalued, but they bring independence, peace, and comfort. So much of what people need is basic, hands-on, and low-tech. It goes unnoticed and takes place quietly, in the privacy of clients' homes and behind closed doors. It is seldom witnessed, but intensely felt by those in their care."

I've never met someone like Judith, an intellectual powerhouse, an accomplished scholar, a corporate executive, and, up there on the stage, a commanding presence. Yet she's also completely down-to-earth, humble, approachable, straight-talking, and authentic. Cosmopolitan, open-minded, and at home in the world (she calls herself a "global citizen"), she is quiet, thoughtful, and serious – even introverted – and also grandmotherly, playful, and charming. I wonder to what extent nursing is an expression of her religious beliefs. Perhaps for Judith Shamian, nursing is her way to fulfill *tikkun olam*, the Jewish imperative to repair the world. Her purpose is no less serious, her vision that encompassing. Some people view the world through a microscope, others with a telescope, but Judith's wide-ranging vision and capacious mind takes in the details as well as the big picture, the individual *and* society at large. She looks to the future while staying firmly rooted in modern nursing values and ancient Jewish ones, too.

After her speech, Judith receives a standing ovation. Then, an attractive, energetic lady with bright red hair and a Newfoundland accent, Lynn Power, who is chair of the national board, bounds up onto the podium to lighten the mood by leading the crowd in a stretch break and a singsong of her rendition of "My Bonnie Lies Over the Ocean": "My body lies over the sofa. My body watches too much TV." These people have fun – especially the Maritime contingent. (In fact, one of the executives from Nova Scotia had so much fun last evening that today she's in a wheelchair with a sprained ankle. I've been bring-ing her ice packs from the kitchen.) Their lively spirit is infectious.

I'll have what they're having.

They make good sense and I love being around their enthusiasm. I'm definitely warming up to Judith's offer, but I'm holding back, still thinking it over – perhaps over-thinking it? My instinct tells me to go for it. There could be some sweet perks to this gig. I'd get to travel, see the country, stay in hotels with big, fluffy white towels and those tiny bottles of shampoo and conditioner – maybe I could even order room service? What fun! And it's not like I have any other commitments or projects on the go at this time. Yes, the timing might be just right to start something new.

A whoosh of pure energy flies at me. It's a tiny package of a woman with bright blue eyes, curly hair, and an impish grin. She's just hurtled out of the bathroom and plowed straight into me. She grabs onto my arm to steady me as I stumble, trying not to fall.

"The hand dryer almost blew me away! You have to take a strong stance in there, or you'll be blasted into outer space," she exclaims.

Who *is* this person?

They'd told me I'd recognize Nurse Jackie Wells. She's a "force of nature," one executive said. "The goddess of community supports," a nurse manager called her.

"What d'you wanna know?" Jackie asks as she sits across from me at lunch. We've loaded our plates at the buffet, breezed past the many people who called out to her and wanted a piece of her, and have finally taken a seat at a table at the back of the ballroom. "Ask away," Jackie says with a huge, inviting smile. "I'm an open book." She spreads the heavy cloth serviette on her lap and picks up her fork.

"For starters, what is 'community support' and what does it have to do with nursing?"

Jackie puts down her fork. "Here's the first thing you need to know," she says. "Home can be a mansion or a log cabin, a teepee, a yurt, under a bridge, or over a sewer or subway grating." Hardly pausing for a breath, Jackie moves on. I put my plate to the side; I don't think Jackie is going to eat at all. "Second, everyone needs a home and wants to be at home. People do not want to be in hospitals or institutions. Third thing: nurses can't do it all. Nursing is not only about nurses."

"It's not?" I guess I'm one of those nurses who thinks it is, who likes to do it all.

"Some of the best nursing care is given by family members, a volunteer, or a neighbour who's willing to travel the journey with the family."

I feel as if I have to "listen fast" to keep up with Jackie's lightning-bolt mind.

"In the hospital, do we ever ask people what they want, and if we do ask them, do we really want to hear their answer? If I worked in a hospital today, I'd challenge that. In the community, it's my job as your nurse to ask that question and mean it. If we can't do it ourselves, we have to bring in people who can. I went into one home. There must have been twenty cats roaming around, no running water. Dirty, dirty, dirty. Every nursing instinct in me told me to take a mop and bucket and get to work. 'He shouldn't be at home,' my manager said. 'Try to bring him to the hospital, Jackie.' But to him, that was his *home,* where he wanted to be. I put old mattresses on the floor in case he fell out of bed. Neighbours checked on him daily. Now, that's nursing. You won't find it in any textbook."

There's no time to ask another question, as Jackie has segued into another story.

"There was a farmer who used to catheterize himself. Kept his catheter woven into the brim of his hat. Out in the field, he'd stop, use the catheter and put it back on his hat. He had to go into the hospital for surgery, picked up some superbug, got a bladder infection, and died there." Jackie's fork, laden with Greek salad, suspended mid-air, doesn't make it to her mouth. "Home care is about caring for people where *they* are, without bias or imposing our values on them. You won't get that in the hospital, and that's what people want. If someone told me I had to eat dinner at five o'clock and shower by eight, I'd pretend I didn't hear them. I'd want to spit at them."

"That's a common scenario in the hospital."

"Let's say you're a proud veteran who's served in the war and fought for our country and now someone tells you, 'Take your pills, dearie.' We are the boss of you. We decide when you can move your bowels and when you can't. It's inconvenient for the staff if they have a bowel movement at change of shift, am I right?" I nod. *This is so true.* "Now, imagine that's your loved one. Once you do that, it becomes clear to you that the hospital takes away your independence and dignity. That's why I love palliative care. Nothing brings you closer to another person than caring for them when they're dying. It's not something every nurse can do or even wants to."

Food for thought. Just as well because I can't eat. Listening to Jackie commands my full attention.

"I could never work in a hospital. Early on, I realized I couldn't give the kind of care I wanted to give in a hospital. In the hospital, everyone's so caught up worrying about getting sued, but should that be the rationale for our nursing care? I would challenge that. The whole place is run by conformity and fear of litigation."

Paradoxically, it was Jackie's most memorable experience that made her leave bedside nursing.

"This cantankerous old coot living out in the middle of nowhere was diagnosed with metastatic bone cancer. 'Okay lady, sit down. I've got something to say,' he told me. 'Number one: if you're here to put me in the hospital, you can get back in that little car of yours and go home. I'm staying right here. Second: I want to have some fun.' Now, I'm a fun-loving person myself, so every visit, I made sure we had fun. He'd never been in a hospital. Born in that house, grew up there. He'd never complain of pain because he was afraid it meant he wouldn't be able to stay home. One day, the house was dark. I could smell impending death. The wife went outside to be with her horse because that gave her comfort. I set to work and gave him a bath, listened to his chest, gave him morphine, checked his bowels. Then I asked him, 'Hank, if I could do one thing for you, what would it be?' He turned to me. There was a sparkle in his eyes. 'Jackie, jump in bed with me.' With my stethoscope around my neck, I lay down beside him and held him in my arms. He cried and I cried and it felt good. His wife walked in and hugged us both. It was a wonderful moment because caring was what this was about. He needed me to be me. That's what made me more dedicated to nursing and also made me leave nursing. I wanted to teach nurses to challenge the status quo, to have the courage to break rules when necessary. I wanted to show volunteers how they can lessen the burden on nurses and family caregivers. People want to help, but they don't know how and we don't let them in." She picks up her fork. "So, that's what I do. Or did. I'm retiring." Finally, she digs into her salad. "There. That'll give you something to chew on for awhile."

"They warned me about you, Jackie," I tease her. She beams, proud of her "bad" rep as a "troublemaker." "They told me, 'There's mischief wherever Jackie goes. When Jackie wakes up in the morning and her feet hit the floor, Satan says, 'Oh no, she's awake.'"

Next, I meet Nurse Andrew Ward, another high-energy person who is the manager of a vast VON site that includes this very area around

Windsor. We grab a corner of the packed lobby to sit and chat. He closes his eyes to concentrate, then opens them wide. "VON is a very kick-ass organization. They welcome creative solutions. We have an innovative day program, assisted living for seniors, and a nursing station on Pelee Island that's run by an awesome nurse. We've started a school nutrition program. Yup, we're feeding hungry school kids. Oh, and a video medicine network and a chronic pain clinic. You'll have to come and see it for yourself," he says. "Gotta run." He hustles off to – what else? – a meeting.

Steve and Anne volunteer for VON by delivering home-cooked meals to people who are unable to shop or prepare nutritious food for themselves.

"Meals and hugs," clarifies Anne.

Diabetic, wheat-free, vegetarian. All kinds of meals. Each day of the week, they volunteer for a different charity. Once, Anne made a thousand cabbage rolls for her church.

We sit in comfy chairs in the hotel lobby. As Anne tells me about what drives them both to be such active volunteers, Steve watches her lovingly. In 1978, Anne escaped to Canada from Czechoslovakia, fleeing a repressive dictatorship. Life was hard for many years, until they met each other and found love. Things are good now, and their gratitude is expressed in their drive to help others. They hold hands and snuggle in close to each other like newlyweds.

Steve explains their shared outlook on life. "Back in the seventies, there was a philosophy called the 'power of positive thinking.' Whatever happens, good or bad, you only find what you're looking for, so look for the positive."

I ask them the secret to their long relationship, and Steve is quick with his answer.

"A person you hate, you only have to tell them once. Someone you love, you have to tell them – and show them – every single day." He gazes at Anne, adoration in his eyes. "We never fight. Oh, arguments, sure, but we always make it right. Because we want to. Another thing.

Make sure you thank your spouse for one thing every night before you go to bed," he suggests, and I take his advice to heart.

Perhaps I will return to Windsor to see Anne and Steve again and bask in their loving presence, to feel the passion between them – and to taste one of those cabbage rolls.

One by one, Judith has lined up these twenty-minute "speed dates" with key people in VON. Our informal "meetings" are held here in the comfortable hotel lobby.

"Come visit us in Thunder Bay," Joan Wekner invites me. She's the nurse manager of the vast Northern Ontario region, plus the prairie provinces of Manitoba and Saskatchewan. I take an immediate liking to Joan and her funky clothes, skull ring, and purple highlights, like mine.

"I've always wanted to go to Thunder Bay," I tell her. (I've had a secret fascination with Thunder Bay ever since an old American boyfriend once asked me how the city got its name. I said, "New York was taken," and it became a private joke that always made us break out in giggles.)

"Working together with the Ministry of Natural Resources, we provide fire line nursing," Joan explained. "When there's a forest fire, we set up base camp – it could be a hotel room, a trailer, or a tent – and treat injuries or stabilize and transfer out. We teach bear safety and conduct stress debriefing sessions. It's not for every nurse. We had one gal from Toronto." She stops for a chuckle. "She complained there was no place to plug in her blow dryer. You have to know what you're getting into, and it helps if you like being out in the bush. I'll arrange for you to go out with Joanna on her rounds. She's sixty-five, still working full-time and incredibly energetic. Joanna provides health care to First Nations' people on the Anishnabe tribe reserve. Sometimes she drives hours and hours to get to people. You should see all the dents in her windshield from gravel roads and highways. Joanna is salt of the earth, what VON is all about. You gotta meet her. When you come, bring warm clothes."

I meet Janice Bernard-Bain, a home care nurse who works in a rough, downtown Toronto neighbourhood known for its poverty, gangs, and high crime rate. None of that fazes Janice. "I see everyone as an individual who needs care." She has a no-nonsense, take-no-prisoners manner with her clients that conveys respect and affection.

"It begins when I make that first call to a client and introduce myself on the phone. That's when our relationship begins and trust is forged. Once, I was covering for a nurse who was sick. 'Where's my regular nurse?' the client asked. 'Your nurse is resting,' I told him. 'You're going to have to love me today.' Yes, with some clients, I speak in that informal way. Some nurses can be too lofty, using jargon or acting aloof. In home care, you have to know how to relate to people. In the hospital you can just pull the curtain and start doing things to them. In home care you have to be good at relationships. You have to want it."

This nurse is impressive, and I'd like to see her in action on the job.

Next, I meet Angela Cross, who is a home care worker, one of those "invisible people" that Judith spoke about. At tonight's closing banquet, Angela will receive a Gold Award for exemplary care of residents in an assisted-living facility. She joins me in the lobby accompanied by her husband, who is a dead-ringer for Elvis Presley with his black, slicked-back hair, white hip-hugging jeans, and sequined jacket. It turns out he's a professional Elvis impersonator. When Angela joins me on the couch, I get a whiff of her perfume, a soft fragrance like velvet peaches. "Elvis" sits beside her and puts his arm around her protectively.

"I'm just a home care worker," she says. "I don't do much, but I love my work and I love my clients." For years, Angela had worked in an accounting firm, but decided it wasn't for her. "I enjoy numbers and I'm good with them, but I missed working with people."

Four years ago, Angela's father got cancer and she was determined to care for him at home. "One day he was in terrible pain and I had to take him to the hospital. I'll never forget the look of relief on his face after he got a shot of morphine. The doctor wanted to admit him but Dad wanted to go back home. 'I'm taking him home,' I told the doctor.

I was so scared to stand up to a doctor, I was trembling. Dad's condition was deteriorating and I didn't know if I could manage to care for him at home, but I wanted to try."

Angela is five foot – if even – has a sweet face, and a gentle demeanour. She looks like a pushover, but clearly is not.

"One day at home my dad said, 'I want to go home.' 'You *are* home,' we kept telling him. I panicked, thinking he was losing it. 'That home,' he pointed upward. A day later, after a peaceful night, he died. It felt holy, like Christmas morning. We weren't happy but we weren't sad. He wanted to be at home and, thankfully, I could provide that for him. It gave me peace knowing I'd fulfilled his wishes. That's why I became a home care worker. I'm not a real nurse, but I'd like to become one, one day."

If that's not real nursing care, what is?

Her husband puts his arm around her. He looks like he's about to break out in song and croon "The Wonder of You."

Just as I'm starting to get the impression that home care is all about death and dying, I meet Suzanne D'Entremont from Yarmouth, Nova Scotia, who's bursting with vitality and enthusiasm about, of all things, "central lines." A central line is an invasive and risky intravenous line placed into a large, deep vein in the body, some that lead directly into the heart. They are routinely used in the hospital, but because of the specialized care they require and risks they involve, I never would have believed they could be used at home.

"Yes," Suzanne says, "our home care nurses care for many clients with central lines. They give chemo and other IV meds, change dressings, and even manage chest tubes, in peoples' homes." She gives me her card, flashes me a huge grin, then pulls me in for a big hug. "Come down east for a visit. We'll show you a good time."

Next is Bonnie Schroeder, whose name tag says "Director of Caregiving."

"*Caregiving*," I say, with a touch of sarcasm. "Isn't that what we all do? Aren't we all caregivers?" I settle into the comfy chair, but Bonnie sits bolt upright. She is quick to correct my misunderstanding.

"No, Tilda. You are a *professional* caregiver. A registered nurse. You are educated and highly skilled. You chose this profession and are paid for your services. When you leave at the end of your shift, the responsibility is off your shoulders. You get breaks, benefits, and a paid vacation. I'm talking about caregivers who are friends, family, neighbours, and volunteers, caregivers who are *conscripted* – even coerced – into this role by love or duty."

I get the feeling she's had to explain this before. However, I should know this. I was once a family caregiver, and a child caregiver at that.

"Family caregivers do the heavy lifting. They save the health care system millions of dollars, but think how hard it is even if you *want* to do it."

How well I know. From the age of six, I helped my father care for my mother, who was physically and mentally unwell. As a child, I was a dutiful caregiver; as an adolescent, a distracted, unhappy one. As a young adult, shouldering the responsibility by myself after my father's death, I became bitter and resentful. Then I became – what else? – a nurse.

I immediately identify with Nicole White, who, like me, was a critical care nurse who once had no interest in home care. She runs an adult day program (ADP) in Corner Brook, Newfoundland, a small fishing outport with a population of twenty thousand. The ADP offers a break, or "respite," as they call it, for family members of people who have Down syndrome, dementia, autism, or mental health issues. "You don't hear of Alzheimer's improving, but in a stimulating environment such as we provide, I've seen it happen," Nicole says, her dark eyes shining. "Giving caregivers respite improves family life, even saves marriages. I love my work and feel I've found my true calling."

Next on the roster is Morag McLean, whose title is "People in Crisis Nurse." She works in Edmonton women's shelters, where she encounters women who have been choked by their partners during episodes of domestic violence or as a sexual game. Morag has developed a scientific protocol to help identify strangulation victims. It's startling to hear about something so horrific from Morag, a gentle, soft-spoken but intense

woman. She remains composed as she talks about this shocking phe-
nomenon that often goes undetected and is more widespread than commonly believed.

"Hands can be weapons that are always at hand. Literally. It doesn't
take a lot of strength – even a child is capable of it." She tells me about
a ten-year-old boy whose father enlisted his help to strangle his step-
mom. The father blamed the murder on his son.

"The first time I was alerted to this problem was when I noticed a
woman who was speaking in a raspy voice, and the whites of her eyes
were blood-red. When she drank coffee she was having difficulty
swallowing. I've since learned that these are classic signs of choking
or strangulation." Morag explains that she purposely uses those two
words interchangeably because "sometimes a woman doesn't respond
to one word, but does to the other. And they'll never volunteer that
information. You always have to ask if you have even the slightest suspicion, and they'll often downplay it."

"So what did you do when you made those observations?"

"She let me examine her and I found striations along her neck, and
bruises. She told me it was only a game. But it's a lethal game," Morag
says grimly. She tells me about a study published in the *Journal of
Emergency Medicine* that found that the risks of attempted murder
increase sevenfold for women who have been strangled by their partner. Forty-four per cent of attempted murder victims had been strangled by a partner. "These findings give us hope that with early detection
and intervention, we might save lives."

I tell her I'd like to visit her and learn more about the work she does.

"You are welcome to come, but just know that if you're the type of
nurse who wants to fix people and find quick solutions to their problems, you'll be disappointed. It's a long process without a lot of
immediate signs of success or progress. Great maturity is required as
well as the ability to take in the whole picture, not just deal with
moment-to-moment needs. These are women who have experienced
domestic violence and abuse. You have to actively create trust and

safety – a nurse can't hide. Often there's no resolution, goals, or signs of progress. What you're doing is planting seeds."

She's a gardener, planting seeds. In the ICU, we see immediate results from our actions and I've always liked that. Could I put in such hard work and not reap a harvest?

Dr. Ariella Lang explains that KT (which I'd mistakenly heard as "KD," which, as any kid knows, is Kraft Dinner) stands for "knowledge transfer," meaning the process of implementing research findings into practice. She is researching the topic of client safety at home. "Medication errors, for example," Ariella says. "We know they happen in the hospital, but they are also occurring in homes, too. We don't know the incidence of medication errors made by family members or unregulated workers, or what interventions could be implemented to reduce them."

"They can't be doing a worse job than we're doing," I say ruefully, alluding to the alarming incidence of medication errors in hospitals, as widely reported in the media.

"Another area I am studying is bereavement support after the death of a loved one."

"Do you mean palliative care?"

"No, I'm referring to the support that families and loved ones need after the death."

"Goodbye and good luck" is our send-off to grieving families. We then turn our attention to the next incoming train wreck. No bereavement care for the families, nor for us.

"You'll learn about the ways grieving people can be supported when you visit VON's bereavement programs in Nova Scotia."

In the evening, at the closing banquet, there's a celebratory meal and entertainment by "Elvis," Angela's husband. Near the end of the gala, they have a surprise retirement celebration for Jackie, who truly looks surprised and is touched to the point of tears. In a glittering, bejewelled tiara and with a hot-pink feathered boa around her neck, Jackie takes the podium to receive flowers and a plaque, and make a farewell speech. She starts off with a few fond reminiscences of her years at VON, where she'd had the "best times of my life."

Jackie was a new, young nurse in a remote, rural posting in the Middlesex region of southern Ontario when she started with VON. "I was so naïve back then. I didn't think I was even allowed to say 'Middlesex.' I could never bring myself to say Middlesex without blushing." The crowd laughs along with her as she goes on to recount a madcap story involving a burst jar of olives in her suitcase, the briny smell that followed her everywhere, the subsequent heap of laundry, and an eventful trip to the laundromat — admittedly, a silly story, but with her animated delivery, the crowd is in stitches.

She's so youthful. It's hard to believe she's retiring. I'm not ready to retire — far from it — but I could take a sabbatical to go on this adventure, which now, after meeting so many enthusiastic people doing such interesting work, seems more like an incredible opportunity that I couldn't possibly turn down than the dull imposition it seemed at first.

After the banquet on Sunday evening, I sit with Judith in an empty boardroom at a long table upon which is a bonsai tree, a large candy dish filled with mints, and a goldfish in a glass bowl with plastic seaweed and a fake pirate's treasure chest. The conference is over; everyone is leaving in the morning. Judith is flying to Ottawa, then Washington, then New York City. I'm heading home to my husband, kids, dog, cat, and job, in Toronto.

"Have you thought about my offer?" Judith asks. "What have you decided?"

It's crunch time. These few days at the AGM have been so pleasant, but I haven't kicked my ICU habit. I'll go back, I tell myself, after the four months this assignment will take. Denise, my manager in the ICU, has always accommodated my "creative scheduling" habits. I'm sure she'll let me take some time off work, and still squeeze in shifts whenever I'm in town. I'm not completely sold on this project, but I am drawn to Judith, intrigued by her. Though I'm not going to drink the Kool-Aid, I am curious to see what she sees and figure out why she – and everyone I've met – is so passionate about all of this.

I watch the goldfish swimming around and around in its bowl.

That's its home. Seeing that little fish, happy at home, reminds me of many patients over the years who used their final breaths to communicate their last wish – to "go home."

Okay, I'll do it, I tell her, but on one condition. I won't be bound by VON's agenda or restricted by only what they can offer me. I want to learn everything – or as much as I can – about health care that takes place beyond the hospital walls.

Judith accepts my condition and looks pleased with my answer.

A sabbatical, I tell myself; that's what this will be. Just dip my toe in, test the waters. Anyway, how hard could it be? It's a piece of cake, easy as pie – and other pastries, too.

4

OUTDOORS

USUALLY, NOT MUCH HAPPENS in the month of August, but in mid-July, I receive the itinerary of my first visits, to start August 1st. The rest of my trip will continue in September. I will be spending two separate days with home care nurses: one in Hamilton – a medium-sized, working-class city an hour west of Toronto – and the second in Toronto, where I live. I'll join each nurse on their rounds, and if the clients give consent, I'll sit in on the visit and observe.

In the Hamilton VON, at eight a.m. sharp, I meet Nurse Chelsea, eager to show and tell me all about home care nursing. She's been a nurse for only a year, but is knowledgeable and self-assured. Adorable, too, with wide-set eyes, clear skin, a petite figure in a sky-blue coat over VON navy pants and white shirt. Chelsea launches into the now-familiar refrain.

"In school, they warned us, 'Don't go into home care. You'll lose your skills.' But what skills do you have when you graduate? None." I sit beside her in her compact car while she organizes her day and figures out her route, deferring cases with infection-control issues to the end of the day to prevent spread.

At the first house we check a client's blood sugar and give a shot of insulin, then the same at the next stop. It seems strange. "At home, don't clients give their own meds?"

"Some people aren't able and some don't want to." Chelsea tries to hide the disapproval we both feel. Nurses always believe our role is to foster independence and self-care.

Chelsea pulls into the driveway of a tiny bungalow with a clothes-line and garden gnomes on the front lawn. "I've been training Apollina to give her husband's insulin. Let's see where's she's at with that today."

In a dark living room with lacy doilies on every surface, a burgundy shag rug, and heavy oil paintings depicting Jesus as a Greek Orthodox icon, Apollina sits beside her husband on the couch. She timidly pricks his finger and tests his blood sugar with the glucometer while he stares blankly at the TV set, which isn't even on. Apollina hesitantly but competently draws up insulin into a plastic syringe and gives him a shot in his abdomen. Throughout it all, Chelsea supervises closely and gives them both constant encouragement.

As we get ready to leave, Apollina accompanies us to the door. "Tomorrow? You come tomorrow?"

"Tomorrow's my day off," Chelsea says gently. "Another nurse will come."

Apollina is miffed. She asks for Chelsea's home phone number and looks surprised when Chelsea won't give it to her. "But we're friends, no?"

"I'm your nurse," Chelsea says. "I can't give you my number. It's policy."

"Policy?" Apollina looks puzzled, like she doesn't know what the word means, then dismissive, as if surely *policy* doesn't apply to them. "You want coffee? I make for you." We thank her but get up to go. I follow Chelsea to the door. Apollina grabs my arm and holds me back. Her fingers find a rip in the sleeve of my jacket. She fondles it as if to say, *If you stay awhile, I'll fix this for you.*

We feel her fear and loneliness. It's difficult to leave her, but we must; Chelsea has another client to see. Apollina follows us outside and watches us from the side of the house, where she stands rearranging

laundry hanging on a clothesline. I can feel her eyes on us as Chelsea
backs out of the driveway and turns onto the street.

"I'll arrange for them to have more home care visits," Chelsea tells
me. "They're not yet ready to go solo."

We drive for a few minutes, then pull into the parking lot of a strip
mall opposite a grimy, four-storey, pre-war building. As we cross the
street, a bus roars by, splashing us with dirty rainwater. "One of the
hazards of this job," Chelsea says, wiping off the bottom of her coat.

The smell of sad cooking hits me as we enter the building – it's
cabbage or potatoes, or both, but to me, it's the smell of poverty and its
residue of despair. On the third floor, an apartment door stands ajar.
Just before we go in, Chelsea warns me: "You'll want to take in a huge
breath of air before we go in because once we're inside, you won't want
to do much breathing. Breathe though your mouth."

We enter a dim room and are hit with a wave of heat that seems to
intensify the pervasive musty, sour, unwashed smell – that does indeed
make me hesitant to breathe it into my body. Laszlo, a painfully thin man
who looks much older than his fifty-four years, is lying in bed covered
with a brown and orange crocheted blanket. Two cats sit like bookends,
at his head and feet. A different, but equally unpleasant smell hits me in
the hallway, where I step out to get away from the bedroom's stench. This
stink is emanating from the bathroom, lit only by a night light. The
bathtub is filled with well-used kitty litter for the two cats, plus two
more I spotted, one stalking a fake fur mouse and the other nibbling cat
food from a bowl on the floor beside the toilet. *That makes four.*

Back in the bedroom, Laszlo had been watching a chef prepare a
bouillabaisse on the Food Channel, but turned it off when Chelsea
arrived. They are chatting and he looks so much happier than when we
first arrived. Chelsea is here to irrigate his urinary catheter, which is
draining sluggishly due to sludge and sediment. Without irrigation,
the catheter could become blocked. Chelsea opens a closet where the
medical supplies are stored and out pops another cat. *Five.* Using a
footstool as a procedure table to lay out the sterile syringe and bottle

of saline, Chelsea gently performs this simple procedure. My ICU instinct prompts me to want to measure the urine and to wonder about his hourly output, but I remind myself that such close tracking of ins and outs is not necessary at home. It's hard to make the switch. In the ICU, I know each time my patient coughs, along with the amount, consistency, and colour of phlegm; out here, I might not know if my patient even had a cough.

Laszlo has ALS and can move very little. In an hour, a home care worker will come to give him a bed-bath, get him up into a wheelchair, and feed him. He waves a cheery goodbye as Chelsea packs up to go. "Work smart, not hard," he calls out to her.

That's exactly how Chelsea does work, constantly updating her schedule on her phone, calling ahead to make sure the next client is ready for her.

What a relief to get outdoors, away from the heat and smells. "It's August and it felt like the furnace was on. It was like a Bikram yoga studio in there."

"You'll find a lot of people keep the heat cranked up," Chelsea says.

Next, we meet Mina, whose home is also overheated and close with repellent odours. Mina is a morbidly obese diabetic whose mobility is restricted due to her massive size and swollen arms and legs. She sits on a couch in track pants and an oversized sweatshirt covered in matted pills. Her legs are inflamed and dripping with infected fluid. With such a protruding stomach, there is no way Mina would be able to reach them herself to apply ointments, dressings, and pressure bandages. Her husband, Al, who's sleeping off a hangover, takes care of Mina unreliably. Chelsea suggests leg exercises to improve circulation and Meals on Wheels because grocery shopping is difficult for them and their diet is poor. Mina speaks Portuguese and little English, so conversation is limited.

As Chelsea starts to clean and wrap Mina's legs, Mina complains of pain in her big toe. "*Dolore, dolore*," she moans, pointing to the place where her right big toe once was, where there is now an empty space. Her toe was amputated due to gangrene. It's phantom pain, Chelsea explains, though pain, nonetheless. After treating her legs, Chelsea checks to make sure that Mina has a sufficient supply of painkillers on hand.

"Yeah, yeah," Al mutters. He's up now and busy cooking in the kitchen. "Give her some of those number threes of Tylenol," he hollers.

The smell of frying meat wafts in, making me instantly queasy. Al is cooking lunch for their blind dog, Taser. I watch from the living room as Al pours half a bottle of barbeque sauce into the frying pan. "Would *you* like dry chicken with no sauce? I think not."

Back in the car, Chelsea says, "In some homes you may see behaviours that you disapprove of, but you don't want to lecture or impose your values onto your clients. If people choose to live a certain way, what right do we have to change it? You have to always remember, you are a guest in their home. You have to tread lightly."

"We face the same issues in the hospital when people's lifestyle choices affect their health or if they don't take care of themselves, but we have a lot more leeway to try to bring them in line. Afterall, there, they're on our turf. They go by our rules."

"In their home, we respect theirs. It's whatever they say."

"In the hospital, it's what *we* say." I realize that now.

But one thing I've learned: Complex decisions about health care spending and about the burden that people's personal behaviours place on society should never be conducted at the bedside – or on an individual basis. They are best left to public debate and policy development.

Watching Chelsea at work does make me realize something: in the hospital, we talk a lot about "patient-centred care," but now I see what PCC actually looks like. In the hospital, we still have a long way to go to create a culture that puts patients first, that is truly patient-centred, not doctor-, nurse-, or technology-centred.

As we drive to our next stop, I notice something else that's different about home care nursing; you're not in the hospital. Not to be in the hospital feels completely different – liberating and soothing. Best of all, you're *outdoors*, which feels wonderful, because no matter how smoggy, polluted, or humid city air may be, it's fresher than hospital air.

Another thing. Yes, Chelsea is efficient, but she's not rushing in, getting the job done, and racing out. She stops to talk with her clients, not just about their health but their families and their interests, too. Everything she did for Laszlo, and then for Mina, she did while talking with them, asking questions, and observing closely. And there's no swagger, no bravado, and none of the forced cheeriness many well-meaning hospital nurses offer to placate or cajole patients. I never realized how brisk and authoritative we can be in the hospital until I heard the slow, calm way Chelsea spoke to Laszlo, and saw how unhurriedly she opened the irrigation kit, draped a sterile field, took down the covers, exposed his penis, cleaned the meatus, disconnected the catheter, irrigated the bladder, et cetera, all the time touching his body so gently. Believe me, I would have done that little procedure so fast it would make your head spin. In the hospital, we go at one tempo — *prestissimo*. In people's homes, you go at theirs.

At the next house, a man stands at the screen door, waiting for Chelsea.

"Giovanni! What about the pasta we talked about? The ice cream?" Chelsea pretends to scold him. He's lost more weight since undergoing chemotherapy for colon cancer and is very thin. Chelsea asks about his diet, appetite, and energy as she disconnects a small bottle of chemo that had infused into the IV port on his chest. She strikes a balance between the familiarity of pals and the objectivity of a professional. Chelsea takes his vital signs and inquires about his weight loss, bowel movements, nausea, mood, and his wife and her health issues. Giovanni is upset about ten dollars he had to pay for an extra delivery of supplies that another nurse failed to order in sufficient amounts. "It's a lot of money for us."

Chelsea goes out to the car for more supplies and explains, "In the community, we work on a shoestring. Once, I actually used a shoestring — a hockey skate lace — plus duct tape, to bind a hernia. I've used coat hooks to hang IVs and plastic milk jugs for sharps containers."

Guiltily, I think of our hospital stockroom, jam-packed with lots of everything, most of it disposable, along with a laboratory-created product to be applied to every bump, bruise, wound, abrasion, and fissure. (For an ordinary bed-bath we're supposed to use chemical-soaked, antimicrobial-impregnated, pre-moistened "towelettes" instead of plain old soap and water.) In the hospital, we go through supplies as if they are unlimited. We use them liberally, and rarely give a thought to the cost involved or the waste created.

At the next house, Norma, a retired schoolteacher with kidney cancer, has a drain in her abdomen that takes thirty minutes to empty. She hangs her drainage bag on a cupboard door handle to allow gravity to speed up the process. Chelsea takes her blood pressure before and after, both sitting and lying down.

"I love having a nurse visit me," Norma tells me. "Last week at the hospital a young medical student examined me. He was so formal! 'How did your disease present itself?' he asked me. I thought of saying, 'It said, *Hi Norma, it's me, Cancer.*'"

Afterwards, Chelsea and I stop at Tim Hortons. "It's still strange to call patients 'clients,'" I say.

"Think of it this way," she says. "In your own home, you're you, you're not a patient."

She has a point.

We move on. In the moments before we enter each home, I feel apprehensive. There's a way that entering people's homes is as invasive as putting catheters into their bodies or my fingers inside them, things I routinely do in the ICU. Yet each person who opens the door is pleased to see us and welcomes us in.

In between another two visits, I ask Chelsea about home care nurses' wages. They are less than the going hospital wage, but Chelsea likes that VON pays a salary, not a fee-per-visit, like for-profit home care companies. This arrangement gives her more financial stability and means she can stay with her clients as long as necessary, without any pressure to rush and make as many visits as possible to increase her income.

"Let's say you're going in to give an injection, but you see other problems, like skin breakdown, or a burnt-out caregiver. You can't put blinkers on and ignore that. You have to stay and address that. You stay until the work is done."

I can see how that's probably not the best business model, but the perfect nursing one.

Another personal question: "Aren't you lonely working by yourself? I'd miss working with a team."

"The client and the family become your team," Chelsea says, but I'm not convinced.

"What about the socializing, the gossip? Who do you eat lunch with? Shoot the breeze with? Talk with about a complicated situation?"

"We have a daily phone huddle, conference calls, and monthly team meetings in the office, but it's true, out here, you have to be self-reliant. If I listen to someone's chest and it doesn't sound right, it's up to me to know what to do about it."

As for socializing, it is a welcome change to get to talk directly with clients and it's satisfying to be doing things *with* people, not *to* them. In the ICU there are so many procedures and treatments that we perform on our patients that no amount of gentleness or painkillers can mitigate. Often, it seems, our treatments make people feel a lot worse in the hope of making them better. Home care nursing feels more *beneficent* than hospital nursing. And I don't know if it's VON or home care itself, but there is a culture of kindness here that is often lacking in the hospital. A detached attitude, a harsh word, or a lack of basic courtesy would be unacceptable out here. Unfortunately, it is commonplace in the hospital.

We have seen a lot of people over the day – ten patients in eight hours, which included time for driving, parking, telephone calls, and charting. In fact, I learned they leave the client's chart in their house and encourage the client to read it and make their own notes in it. In the hospital, you have to make an appointment with a senior administrator for permission to view your chart and can only do so in their presence.

"We're not as tied to the computer as you are in the hospital," Chelsea says.

"Tell me about it. Computer charting often takes me away from my patients."

Chelsea takes pride in her relationships with clients. "I'm sure I could work faster if I didn't stop to chat, but it means so much to them and to me, too."

"In the ICU you can be a decent, safe, and competent nurse, know everything about a patient's medical problems, but nothing about them as a person."

"In home care, that wouldn't fly. Knowing the client is part of your care. You have to want that connection and be good at relationships."

I wonder what it would be like to work in this gentle, slower-paced environment, rather than the full-tilt pressure cooker of the hospital.

"I love home care," Chelsea says. "Every day, I'm so excited to see my clients."

"I gotta tell you, you'd be hard pressed to hear a hospital nurse say that."

Our last stop of the day is to see a client who lives in a subsidized housing complex. It's an old building with creaky plumbing and infused with the pungent smells of exotic spices. We stand out in the dimly lit hallway, knock on the door, and wait for Anwar, Chelsea's client. A toilet flushes and water and waste gurgle through the pipes. Eventually Anwar opens the door. Before entering, we slip off our shoes and add them to rows of other pairs of shoes outside the door. Anwar is shivering, wrapped in a blanket, a full urine bag dragging along the floor. He doesn't say a word, and we both become alarmed when he stumbles across the room and slumps down to the floor to lie on his prayer rug. Chelsea takes his temperature while I take his pulse and blood pressure. He is too weak to talk, only managing to say, "Thank you for the very good care." Anwar has leukemia, so Chelsea knows he could go into septic shock very quickly. She calls an ambulance and we wait until it arrives to take him to the hospital.

"His wife left him," Chelsea tells me. "Here they are, alone in a foreign country, with a six-month-old baby, and he's so ill. She couldn't cope and went back to her family in Nigeria."

"In the hospital, we see only their illness. You see their lives."

It was a great day. For such a young nurse, Chelsea is wise. I learned a lot from her.

For my second assignment, I get to spend a day in Toronto with Janice, the home care nurse from the AGM. I remember her strong hands, lustrous brown skin, perfect teeth, and, most of all, the forthright, lighthearted way she described her client interactions. Her territory is a sketchy neighbourhood, one I don't usually frequent. It's often in the news for all the wrong reasons: gun violence, racial tensions, gang warfare. Janice thinks the media profiling worsens the problem. "The real problem is poverty, because that leads to poor health, despair, loss of dignity, and resorting to crime to survive and drug addiction to numb the pain."

Janice's first client is an eighty-year-old Chinese man who has dementia. A daughter stands off to the side of the living room, staring at us warily, while the son and father sit on the couch. The room has little in it, other than the couch and TV. The only decoration is a serpent-shaped calendar for the Year of the Snake.

"I like the hospital." The father gives a huge, toothless grin. "I hate it," the son tells Janice. "I'm the one who has to take him."

The father rocks back and forth. The daughter still stands, now scowling at us in a menacing way, not saying a word. The son has folded his arms across his chest and looks away from his father and us.

"I like the nurse at the hospital," the father says. "She's very nice."

"That nurse is okay. I've seen better," the son grumbles.

"It's a party. I like it. I like it."

"Some party," the son mutters.

"This is our first meeting today, so it's just a checkup," Janice explains to them.

"I'm good. Very good," the father says. "No complaints."

"Tell the nurse about the pain, Dad."

"I feel good," the father says.

"But what about your pain? In the night?"

"I feel good."

"He doesn't know what he's saying. He's on his best behaviour for you."

"What do you see as the problem?" Janice asks the son.

"He has these urges. Sexual urges. Cravings, too. For sweets. His blood sugar is up."

The father beams. The son is upset. The daughter stands frozen, staring, unblinking.

"Dad won't do what I tell him," the son says. Janice nods at him while taking the father's blood pressure and listening to his chest with her stethoscope. "Don't bother doing that," he tells her. "His doctor already checked him out." Janice gives him a look over the top of her glasses that silences him momentarily.

She turns her attention to the father. "How are you feeling, Mr. Chung?"

"I love to visit the Princessa Margarita," the father sings out, clapping his hands.

"He means Princess Margaret Hospital. That's where we go for his chemo."

Back in the car, Janice identifies a number of issues of concern that she plans to follow up on, and asks me my impression.

"There's a lot going on there. The family dynamics look complex and the daughter seemed catatonic, possibly paranoid. Well, definitely, not *normal*."

"Normal is overrated," Janice says with a laugh. "Whatever normal is, you don't see much of it. You see a lot of people who have mental health issues. So often they fall through the cracks of the system and don't get the care they need."

I have a feeling that on Janice's watch, no one falls through the cracks.

We drive through the city streets, past Lucky Store, Jimmy's Felafel House, Cash Converters, Pay Day Loans, bingo halls, dollar stores, and a subway underpass covered in graffiti. A Salvadoran restaurant serves *pupusas*, a Korean place offers barbeque, a Filipino storefront arranges "remittances," and an Indian grocery store is doing a brisk business this morning. Janice pulls into a parking lot to call the next client. "No, I haven't forgotten you," Janice assures her. "I still love you. I'm on my way." She turns onto a quiet side street. "You'll meet Louise, a seventy-one-year-old with CML, chronic myeloid leukemia."

"My body is yours." Louise lifts her sweater so Janice can inject a shot of cytarabine, a chemotherapy drug, into her abdomen. Her face is bruised from a fall she had in her kitchen, but she's mobile, very sharp, and still drives.

"Yes, I'd drive with you," I say after chatting with her for a few minutes.

"My husband built this house and I don't want to leave it," Louise tells me. She goes over to play songs for us on a pipe organ. She sings "Cry Me a River" and then "Blue Heaven," her stiff, swollen, arthritic fingers stumbling over the keys. "I'm not ready to lie down, yet," she says, standing on the porch to wave goodbye. "Keep me alive, Janice. I'm not ready to go yet."

"We'll do our best." They exchange an expression that conveys the message, *We're in this together.*

Next, we see a Sri Lankan woman with legs that are inflamed and wet with sores.

"They look painful. Are they?" Janice asks.

The son translates and the mother nods, clasping her hands at Janice in gratitude. She's Hindu, has a grey smudge on her forehead, indicating she'd done *puja*, her morning prayers. The TV plays loudly – a Tamil soap opera – and the air is thick with cumin, fenugreek, and garlic. The sensory overload makes it hard to concentrate on these legs, the reason we're here. To me, they look infected, but Janice explains that the problem is poor circulation. She's set up an appointment with a vascular surgeon and for now is putting a compression dressing on the legs to improve venous blood flow.

The day whizzes by. We see a woman in a retirement home with polymyelitis in her foot, a stubborn wound that resists healing. Janice cauterizes it with silver nitrate.

"You've tried everything, haven't you, Janice, even prayers," the woman says to Janice gratefully.

We meet a man who's living in a rundown and filthy group home who has a number of medical problems, including epilepsy, a gang-related gunshot wound that resulted in a colostomy bag on his abdomen, and abscesses on his arm along the vein he uses to inject drugs. At a previous visit he'd mentioned extreme thirst and that he was losing weight. Janice arranged for him to see a doctor, who diagnosed diabetes. "Until we've got your blood sugar under control, your wound won't heal," Janice tells him, but he barely reacts.

"Is he capable of injecting himself with insulin?" I ask when we're outside.

"I think so," says Janice. She gives a dry laugh. "He's certainly capable of injecting himself with heroin. The question is will he care enough about himself to do it."

The next client is a fifteen-year-old Native girl with tuberculosis who's living in a group home. We're here to check if she's taking her meds. But in the midst of our visit, she gets a text on her phone that makes her jump up. "Oh, I gotta go. My pimp is looking for me."

"Where's your mother?" I blurt out the first of many questions that come to mind.

"My mother?" She gives a laugh and runs out the door, leaving it open behind her.

"This is so wrong. I still drive my fifteen-year-old son to school, make his lunch."

"You see things you can't believe," Janice says. "That young girl has been an alcoholic since the age of twelve. She's been abused by her father and her uncles and has been beat up so many times, it's a wonder she's alive." She sees me struggling to take this in. "I guess you don't get to know much about your patients' lives, do you? That's what I didn't like about hospital nursing."

She must feel I'm in need of a change of subject, so she launches into an amusing story to make me laugh and it works. "When I worked in the hospital, there was one surgeon I always clashed with. One Monday he used number eight gloves. On Tuesday, I handed him a pair of eights and he threw them on the ground. 'I want seven-and-a-half,' he barked. 'You used eight yesterday,' I told him. 'So, what? Are you paying for it?' he asked. 'Yes, Dr. Wong. We all are. Those gloves are ten dollars a pair.' I couldn't stand the waste in the hospital. Ask nurses. We know where the waste is."

At the next apartment building, the elevator is broken, so we walk up the eight floors to get to the next client. As we make our way up, Janice fills me in on a disturbing backstory.

"When I first met Warren he greeted me with, 'You're the nurse? You didn't sound black on the phone. I don't usually open my door to black people.' 'Don't make an exception for me,' I said and turned to leave. He called me back in a panic. I've been taking care of him for six weeks and his attitude hasn't improved. At one visit, he was so rude, his dogs looked apologetic, like, 'Please excuse his bad behaviour.'"

At the last visit, Janice discovered what was really bothering him.

"He kept going on about this 'f-ing shit bag this' and the 'f-ing shit bag, that' and the 'f-ing health care system.' 'There's a lot of f-ing going on today,' I told him, but he kept on cursing. Finally, I said, 'This visit isn't very pleasant. I'm leaving.' I got up to go and suddenly he broke down and cried. He poured his heart out to me. His anger was about the colostomy. He couldn't accept it. 'You must hate me,' he said. 'Of course not,' I told him. 'I've long ago learned not to take anything personally – not everyone has social graces."

"That's putting it mildly." I'm impressed by her tolerance of such bad behaviour.

We move on. It's one-thirty, and so far there's been no mention of lunch. Janice says she never stops for lunch.

"Being in and out of so many places, I never feel my hands are clean enough and I'm still in my uniform."

At the next stop, a husband cares for his wife who's terminally ill with a brain tumour. She lies in a bed in the living room. He turns her every two hours to prevent skin breakdown. He charts her morphine doses and correlates it with her bowel movements because of the constipating effect of narcotics. He milks her catheter tubing to drain drops of urine. Her urometer is covered with a colourful cloth bag.

"What a good idea. We should do that in the hospital. Urine is private."

"I came up with that idea to prevent the cat from biting the bag, right, sweetie?" he says to his wife.

I reach down to pet the cat and she hisses at me. I toss a crinkly ball and she stalks it, moving in for a kill. The husband picks her up and cuddles the vicious little thing. In his arms, she purrs. "You're a real caregiver," I tell him.

"No, she is." He points to his wife, Rosie. "She helped me care for my mother." He points to her picture on the wall. "Now, it's my turn to care for her." He sings while she moans softly, but soon she joins him in song. He turns her and as he lifts her legs, she screams out again. "I remember when you liked me to lift your legs." They look at one another in a moment so intimate I turn away and focus on a sign on the wall – "God is a Senior Citizen" – and a reliquary of the bone of St. Francis of Assisi.

"How are you doing?" Janice asks the husband. "Have you had a break?"

He looks surprised, and touched, but doesn't know how to answer. "I've never been asked that question before." He looks like he's never thought about how he's doing, either.

"We tend to forget about the family caregivers," Janice says softly to me. "The Lord is with you," Janice says to them. "He's looking after you both."

Knowing them as she does, she can say this. I've always admired nurses who know how to sensitively infuse their nursing care with spirituality. I haven't figured that out myself.

At the door, the cat takes a parting swipe at me and I scoot out of the way.

"God bless," the husband says to us both.

When we are in the car, we sit silently for a few moments, until Janice expresses the exact same sentiments that are on my mind.

"When I get old or too incapacitated to take care of myself, I don't ever want my kids to care for me. I tell them: Put me somewhere. If I have dementia I won't know the difference. I won't be hurting, you'll be. Visit if you like, but get on with your lives."

"I tell my family the same thing but they won't listen," I say. Perhaps this is a nurse's view. We only want to be on one side of the bed rails, the carer not the *caree*.

"Everyone says they want to stay at home. Family members suffer guilt when they can't keep their loved one at home, but it's not always feasible. Not everyone can do it."

"I agree. All I want is my lipstick and my dog. Maybe some chocolate pudding," I say.

"My kids know I want my high heels and my leopard prints. That's all I need."

"People don't get nurses' sense of humour. We have to be careful when speaking to non-nurses."

"We do tend to have a different take on things, don't we?"

The day brought so much. If you spend even a few minutes with people in their homes, you can't help but feel a measure of their despair, isolation, loneliness, even desperation. Somehow, if there's a home care nurse like Janice there, you feel there's hope. And at least you're outdoors.

5

SAFE HOME

FALL ARRIVES AND IT'S TIME to set out on the next leg of my journey
to Kingston and Trenton, both cities east of Toronto, along the shores
of Lake Ontario. Looking at a road map, I see that if I make a detour
along the way, I could make a brief stop in the little town of Kemptville
(population: 2,500) to finally meet Audrey McClenaghan, my most
dedicated and loyal reader.

I've always been a writer (the kind of kid who was always scrib-
bling in journals, a practice I still continue), but it's only recently
that I've become a published author. For the past few years, I've been
on an amazing ride, writing books about my life as a nurse, travelling, and speaking to nurses, doctors, other professionals, and the
public at large. I am fortunate to have many readers, all over the
world. However, my most devoted fan by far is Audrey McClenaghan
of Kemptville, Ontario. At seventy-nine, she's been "stalking" me
with fan mail, all handwritten in her quaint, rigidly regular cursive
style, each letter and envelope decorated with stickers – flowers,
balloons, kittens, cupcakes.

I call Audrey on the phone.

"Slow down, slow down," she says in a shaky voice. "Who's calling?"

I tell her again, but it takes Audrey a few more moments to realize who it is, to recover from the shock of hearing from me on the *telephone*, and then to put her hearing aid in place. Once all that is done, she's thrilled to hear from me.

"I'm tickled pink!" she exclaims. "I can't hear. I can't see. I can't stand, can barely walk. I am not long for this world, but my dream has come true. At long last, I hear the voice of Nurse Tilda, the famous author. You must come see me as soon as possible, before it's too late. From Toronto, it's only a five-hour train ride."

Clearly, Audrey's sense of time is from a bygone era.

As we're about to hang up, she says, "I await your visit. There's lots of room in my big house for you to stay with me. Don't dilly-dally. Come soon, the sooner the better. My dying wish is to see you, Nurse Tilda."

I'm on someone's bucket list?

Audrey's letters have always been full of questions about the patients, nurses, and doctors I've written about. Here's a sampling from a recent letter.

How is "Suzanne" who had pulmonary hypertension?
Doing well after a lung transplant.

Is purple your favourite colour?
No, blue.

Your heart surgeon, the famous Dr. Tirone David, is that his real
   name? Is he as handsome as you say?
Yes and yes!

Do you have a live-in nanny?
No.

Is night shift awful?
It's often difficult, but only occasionally awful.

Which is more serious: intensive care or critical care?
They're the same thing.

Each letter contains an update on her health status, questions about me and my books, and, always, clippings from the *Kemptville Advance* or *The Ottawa Citizen* tucked into the envelope, which she indicates by writing "encl." – a short-form now replaced by the paper clip icon to indicate an attachment.

Audrey insisted that I take the train to Kemptville so she wouldn't have to worry about me on the highway, but I need my car for my home care visits afterwards. So, I meet her in the train station, near the platform where the train would have let me off. I don't want to risk getting a reprimand. It's like a real old-time train station, with the big round clock, wooden benches, and even a spittoon. It's easy to identify Audrey. There are only two farmers chatting and a mother with her child waiting to board the train. Then there's a frail-looking woman with white hair, thick, large-framed glasses, and orthopedic shoes who has to be Audrey. She stands slightly stooped, leaning into a walker. Beside her is her "young friend," Debbie, who must be in her forties and who Audrey has told me is like a daughter to her. Audrey is overjoyed to see me, but has an unexpectedly formal air about her, so I don't hug her as I went to do at first. In fact, because of her regal bearing and imperious manner, I'm almost inclined to curtsey. Instead, we shake hands and slowly walk out to the parking lot to her 1978 powder-blue Oldsmobile. It's in mint condition with an odometer reading in the triple digits. After Debbie manoeuvres Audrey into the passenger seat, she gets in behind the wheel. I sit in the back seat. At Audrey's urging, Debbie drives slowly, at a rate that seems not much faster than a walking speed. In this neck of the woods, no one seems to mind slowpoke drivers. All the locals know Audrey. As they pass her car, they call out to her with a friendly wave.

Audrey turns around to me. "See, my madcap scheme to kidnap you and bring you here worked, didn't it?" Her expression is triumphant and gleeful. "Look what a simple, old-fashioned handwritten note can accomplish. It brought you here to me. Emails aren't the same as letters. I don't know anything about emails, only that I don't want any. Would an email have tugged at your heartstrings the way my letters did?"

"Probably not," I concede.

Audrey instructs Debbie to stop at Tim Hortons. "We need to feed the famous author," she says. "There's 'nothing worse than a hungry nurse,' right, Tilda Sue?"

I cringe at hearing my middle name, which I never use, but I stand by the quote from *A Nurse's Story*. No one wants a hungry, tired, distracted, or stressed-out nurse, do they? Good luck finding one who's not. I decline the snack, but Audrey wants a coffee and a doughnut and sends Debbie in to get it.

"Use cream. Not the blue milk."

When Debbie gets back in the car, we wait while Audrey daintily sips her coffee and nibbles at her chocolate doughnut and then is ready to move on. (No cup holders in this vintage model.) She taps Debbie's shoulder. "Let's give Charles Dickens back here a tour." Audrey's old clunker moves like a cruise liner smoothly sailing into various ports of call: her bank, where she keeps all the money she plans to bequeath to her church; the town bakery, where she instructs me to roll down the window so I can inhale the sweet fragrance of sugar, cinnamon, and yeast. Outside St. James Anglican Church, where her pew is fourth from the front on the left, she points out her tombstone in the cemetary. "It's ready and waiting. But no flowers, remember?" She glances pointedly at Debbie.

"Mama Audrey hates flowers," Debbie explains.

We move on to the public library where we meet Jean Kilfolyle, a library volunteer and Audrey's best friend. "This is our sacred place for reading and for our teenagers to hang out after school. Here, we hold meetings of the 'Youngsters of Yore Club,'" Jean says.

When we get to Audrey's quaint, cozy home, she shows me around, room by room, pointing out various treasures – pictures on the wall,

Royal Doulton figurines, and china teacups, all of which have been provisionally divvied up among her friends, neighbours, and caregivers. Together they have made it possible for Audrey to remain at home. However, lately, she's been getting more frail and unsteady, needing more and more care, and that's been a concern to them all.

As we've been sitting and chatting, various people have been coming and going in and out of the house, fussing around Audrey. They've brought trays of food and are warming up casseroles in the oven and setting the dining room table with a white tablecloth, all in preparation for what looks like a festive meal.

"What are we celebrating?"

"A celebrity has come to town!" Audrey claps her hands in jubilation. Then, with utter seriousness, adds, "I wanted you to meet all the supporting actors in our little drama. It will be good material for your book."

I nod. "It really wasn't necessary to put them all to this trouble."

"Oh yes, it was. Good thing you made it here to visit me. I could go any day now."

"She's got it in her head she won't live much longer," Hilda tells me. She's Audrey's main caregiver and had been waiting for us at the house when we returned from the train station. She cajoles Audrey. "You must make it to your eightieth birthday bash."

Audrey shakes her head. "Now that I've met Nurse Tilda, I am ready to go. I want to die now, while I'm still healthy. At seventy-seven, I didn't get to heaven. At seventy-eight, I knocked on the pearly gates. At seventy-nine, I feel fine, but now, I'm afraid, old chum, my time has come." At the kitchen table, she opens a notebook to a list of questions she's prepared for me.

"But I want to hear more about you, Audrey."

"Of course. I expected that. You came here for that exclusive interview." She settles into her chair, ready to field my inquiries. "As my biographer you'll need to know all about me for this little book you're writing."

"Actually, it's about home care. Nursing outside the hospital."

"Oh." Momentarily crestfallen, she quickly perks up and begins her story at the beginning. "I was born in 1933 in this very house. I was a librarian, then a secretary for thirty-six years at the community college. I walked three miles each way to work. Want to know why I retired? Computers. They did me in. My life's big disappointment? My high school graduation was in 1951, but on commencement day the king died and the ceremony was cancelled. They rescheduled but that day was the queen's coronation, so again it was cancelled. They ruined both my special days." She looks put out and sounds peeved.

"At least I hope you made it to the prom," I say gently.

"I've been a good girl. I never drank or smoked. And, in case you're wondering, I never had a boyfriend, never got married, never had sex. Yes, I'm a virgin." As I sit taking in that revelation, Audrey rushes to assure me. "I never missed any of it. My life has been without complications."

"What do you do for fun?"

"Healthy living. My health is starting to fail, so I'm ready to go. I'm seventy-nine, so I must die this year. It's September now, but on February 6th, 2013, I don't want to read 'eighty' in my obituary."

(Coincidentally, she shares a birthdate with Bob Marley. I recently saw a documentary on the legendary reggae musician. I wonder if I should inject that bit of trivia, but decide not. I can't quite conjure up an image of Audrey *jammin', jammin', jammin'.*)

"My eyes and ears aren't good," she says. "I can't walk well."

"By my standards, you're in pretty good shape."

She watches me as I take notes. "Don't describe me as weird, just wonderful."

"May I use your real name, Audrey?"

She arches an eyebrow and gives me a perturbed look. "Whose name were you thinking of using?"

Good point.

Audrey leans back in the deep chair. "Well, now that I've met Nurse Tilda Sue, what more do I have to live for?"

Audrey is ready to die today; she's written her eulogy and has even arranged for her cremation and made her funeral arrangements.

"I ordered a pink container from a catalogue. It's ceramic but it won't break because there's a copper lining. I will weigh four pounds, the cremation guys told me. The hole is just waiting for me to fill it. Six thousand dollars includes getting you to the church and digging the hole. I've got a power of attorney for my personal care and one for my property. All I know is I don't want to end up in your ICU."

"Not many people are as prepared as you, Audrey. I'm impressed. And you seem to have no fear of death. Do you pray, Audrey? Does Jesus give you comfort?"

She gives a contented smile. "No, Nurse Tilda does."

"That's a lot to live up to, Audrey."

Another of Audrey's caregivers, Virginia, joins us in the living room. She's from Chile and is apparently an exotic sight around here, as Audrey notes, "We don't have many dark folk in this town." Virginia pays no notice to her comment and tells me about another client who, at 103, "cooks, bakes, tends her garden. She told the office to stop sending a home care worker, but it's good for her not to be left alone. Children these days are busy or don't make the time. Neglect can kill."

I ask Audrey about the gadget hanging from her neck on a string.

"I would have thought an experienced nurse like you would know all about it. It's my lifeline. If I press this button, they all come running," she says. "I used it only once. 'What's wrong?' they asked. 'My leg went on me,' I told them. 'I've fallen and can't get up.'"

(Yes, those are her exact words.)

Around the table sits Team Audrey: Jean serves us her creamy home-made chicken à la king from a bone china tureen, using a sterling silver ladle, as you would expect from a refined lady whose cats are named "Tea" and "Crumpets." Terry is a teacher from the local college who worked with Audrey. He's brought over a music CD for me. It's a collection of army songs that he has been researching. "The Korean War was the last war when soldiers sang songs that brought them closer as men. Today, soldiers are on their cellphones, talking to loved ones at home." Next-door neighbour Ed tips his hat to me. Ed picks up Audrey's mail, does her banking and grocery shopping, makes home repairs, cuts the grass, checks the furnace, and shovels the snow.

"Audrey, you're an impresario," I tell her. "You bring people together. You make things happen."

"Yes, they do tend to flock 'round me like bees after honey." She bats her eyes at me as if helpless at reigning in her irresistible magnetism.

This must be how life used to be, in the good old days. And it wasn't just about casseroles. There were real connections, communities of neighbours who knew each other and were involved in each other's lives. These days, every summer you hear on the radio, "It's a scorcher today, a heat wave. Make sure to check on elderly or people living alone." The members of Audrey's close-knit entourage don't need such prompts, nor do they need to be organized into shifts, or told what to do. They each show up and simply provide whatever is needed out of genuine care and concern for Audrey. We know it takes a village to raise a child, but it takes one to care for an elder, too. We all need to be part of a village.

At the end of the evening, Jean is the last to go. Audrey and I step out onto the porch to say goodbye. Audrey calls out to her, "Safe home!"

Jean calls back, "Nighty-night, Audrey. Safe home, Nurse Tilda."

I don't recognize the phrase and Audrey explains. "It's an Ottawa Valley saying. It means get home safely."

Before I go upstairs to bed, Audrey gives me a little china bell to use if I need anything during the night and want to call her.

"It's nice for a nurse to have a call bell for a change. Ring all you want. I won't hear a thing."

At seven in the morning, Audrey calls me down to the kitchen. She wants to show me today's vital signs (along with the last few months' worth), recorded herself in that script I've become so familiar with from her letters. Her cursive strokes and loops are as precise and consistent as a computer-generated cursive font.

a.m. blood sugar 7.0
blood pressure 123/65
heart rate 72
temp. Nearly normal

"You see? The entire performance takes place here, at my kitchen table. Vital signs, eye drops, blood sugar. It's also where I compose my epistles to you."

Using her walker, she gets up and carefully makes her way over to a cupboard where she takes out a toy, plastic stethoscope. She places the bell on my chest and pretends to listen to my heart.

"How'm I doing?"

"Your ticker is right as rain," she says. "As for you, you're the cat's meow."

She injects insulin into her thigh, then heads to the avocado-green refrigerator to show me bowls of insulin syringes. They've already been prepared by Hilda and given colour-coded labels. "Red is my Novolog. That's the fast-acting one. White is Humulin R. I take that before meals. Pink is NPH. I take that in the afternoon. I can just barely make out which is which."

Hilda has arrived and is making pancakes and sausages for our breakfast. She leans close to whisper to me, "Audrey's got selective vision. She says her eyesight is going, but I've seen her pick up a black thread off the navy blue carpet. I love her – I treat her like my grandmother – but boy, can she be stubborn."

These observations, Audrey pretends not to hear. Selective hearing, too, perhaps? She knows I'm spying on her but I think she likes it.

As I'm packing up to go, Audrey announces, "I've got the perfect title for your little book."

"Okay. Shoot." I open my notebook and take out a pen.

"*And She Said.*" Audrey sits back, looking pleased.

"What does that mean?" I close my notebook.

"The book is about me, isn't it?"

"No. You may be in it, but it's about home care," I remind her as delicately as possible.

"Oh." Her mouth drops open, she looks crushed.

"I'm sorry, Audrey," I rush to apologize.

"It's nothing dear, it's just that, well, I thought you were writing a book about me so that I can become as famous as thee."

"I explained it to you on the phone and in my letter." *Last night, as well.*

She sits up straight and looks away from me for a moment. "Here I thought you were a celebrity, but I see that you're just an ordinary person." She turns back. "Never mind. At least I had you here for a measly twenty-four hours. Now come back soon. Don't dilly-dally. I don't have forever, you know."

Now that her cheery spirits have returned it seems like a good juncture at which to leave. I'm glad I came to see Audrey and her sweet, protected life. I have a feeling that not all seniors out there are as well cared for as Audrey at home in her rare and precious little world.

6

OASIS

I'M OUT HERE, back out on the road again, enjoying my freedom and this break from the hospital in my new role as roving nurse. After driving an hour from Kemptville, I arrive at VON's Kingston office, where I meet the nurse manager Carol Cooke, who introduces me to Hazel, a volunteer who drives people to their dialysis treatments, waits for them, and gets them home.

"This isn't a visit to the beauty salon," Hazel says gruffly, like she *means business.* "It's a life-saving procedure. Some of the people I drive are very sick." Hazel describes herself as a "serial volunteer." "I've done it all – Beavers, Brownies, Girl Guides, the hospital auxiliary. Volunteering is in my blood. VON covers my gas, parking, wear and tear on my car. In a good week, I can put on as many as five hundred kilometres. And I've dealt with a few crises, too. One person, I took straight to the emergency department. You have to be brave to take this on. It's like sitting by the emergency exit on an airplane, knowing you have to be the one to open the hatch in the event that the plane is going down."

Carol drives me over to the Oasis, an apartment building of about ten floors that has been turned into an assisted-living residence.

Seniors can live independently, in their own surroundings, but have access to various levels of assistance, as needed.

Doris and Henry have been married for seventy-two years and have lived at the Oasis in a one-bedroom apartment for the past few years. Doris has been looking forward to meeting me and is waiting in the basement lounge where there's an old piano, a new computer, and lots of comfortable couches and rocking chairs, many draped with handmade afghans and quilts. She and Henry sit at a card table. Doris is quiet, but Henry is busy conversing animatedly with an old friend that only he can see.

"Here, I get a break from taking care of him," Doris says, rolling her eyes. "I'm completely stressed out, at his beck and call, running hither and yon. Sometimes I wish I could end it, both him and me. Me, especially, I can't take it anymore." I believe her, yet her words are strikingly at odds with her composed presence and prim appearance in a periwinkle-blue cardigan over a lacy white blouse with a cameo brooch at the neck, her pink lipstick, and perfectly coiffed hairdo.

"How long have you been Henry's caregiver?

"Fifty-four years! Ever since I married him. He's a man, right? Today he's angry because they took away his driving licence." Henry does look very agitated.

"Theytookitawayfrommetookitawayfrommetookitaway . . ."

"When did that happen?" I ask him, but Doris answers.

"Seven years ago, but for him, it's like yesterday. The last time he drove he went through a set of red lights. When I politely pointed that out, he asked me, 'I'm driving?'"

"Do you think you would be safe to drive?" I ask Henry.

"I can drive. Whynotwhynotwhynotwhynotwhynotwhynot . . ."

Doris shakes her head. "Thank God he's not on the road," she mutters. "Can you imagine? I envy friends whose husbands are gone." She takes a starched handkerchief from her purse and wipes drool from the corner of Henry's mouth.

She speaks so openly in front of him that she must believe he doesn't understand her, or perhaps doesn't care if he does.

"So, tell me what's stressing you now, Doris."

She shoots me a withering glance. "What annoying questions you ask." Despite her exasperation, she humours me with an answer. "Can't you see he's completely daft? Didn't you notice how he says the same things over and over?" Her glare is piercing; she can't understand why I don't get it. "Not only that, but he thinks I'm poisoning the food and spending all his money." She rolls her eyes at him. "As if he had any. Sometimes, he gets aggressive with me." She stops short and doesn't want to talk more about that. "I'm run ragged from morning until night taking care of him. I have to empty his urine bag. I dress him, feed him, bathe him, shave him. Who do you think cleans him up? I have no time to kick up my heels. I never get to go anywhere nice."

Annoyed with my questions, Doris gets up in a huff and walks off, thus signalling an end to our conversation. I look around at the other residents sitting in the room, to see whom I can speak with next. At that moment, out of nowhere, a group of noisily exuberant women, dressed in red hats and purple scarves, marches into the communal room singing, clapping, and stomping. "When you're happy and you know it, clap your hands . . . stomp your feet." At the end, they give a cheerleader's shout: "Watch out, dementia is catching."

It feels like I'm in an episode of the old sitcom *Golden Girls*. Meanwhile, more Oasis residents have gathered, eagerly waiting to meet me and tell me their life story.

Sam pushes forward in order to be next. "Welcome to our hangout," he says, waving around at the room. "The Oasis is a great place. We all look after each other. There's a ninety-nine-year-old resident who's being looked after by her sixty-year-old son who has dementia and cataracts. The mother is doing better than the son, but we make sure to check in on both of them throughout the day. There's lots of staff available to help you with whatever you need, whenever you need it. We have a monthly bowling outing and a weekly movie night, but we have to be careful which movies we show because of . . ." He looks over at a sweetly smiling, white-haired woman sitting on an over-stuffed recliner with her feet resting on a low stool, a pink crocheted afghan smoothed over her lap. Her seat has been positioned in the centre of the room, so that everyone has to pass by or walk around her. "That's Gwyneth Patterson," Sam says of the woman they protect from risqué movies. "She's ninety-seven and a born-again Christian. A holy roller. We don't want to shock her." Gwyneth smiles at me serenely.

"Yup, this room is well-used and used well." Sam seems to be the self-appointed Oasis social convener. "We have parties, play euchre, meet friends. There are more women than men, so I have my pick. I'm quite the lady's man." Sam leans back in his spaghetti sauce–stained black T-shirt pulled taut over his belly and baggy grey sweatpants. "Yup, you never stop looking, even at our age. But I like to play the field. All the guys here do. There's lots of romances going on. Yup, lots of reasons to get up and get dressed in the morning."

I note that Gwyneth keeps her eye on me, watching my every move as I work my way around the room, conducting my interviews. Ruth, who's been waiting to tell me her story, sits patiently beside Gwyneth, who's observing the passing parade in front of her.

"For twelve years, I cared for my husband at home," Ruth says. "But then he became violent, and I had to put him into a psychiatric facility. Since I've been here, I've lost a hundred pounds. I'd gotten up to three hundred taking care of my husband. It didn't bother me to care for him. He would have done the same for me. But now, it's *my* time. I'm knitting, sewing, doing macramé, and collecting butterflies. My husband used to call me his butterfly. Oh, I love to sew dolls, arrange flowers, make things beautiful – which reminds me, summer's over. Time to bring out the fall decorations. I'm in charge of decor. I'll take down the butterflies and put out lots of gold, red, orange. Butterflies are free, they say."

"Butterflies are an omen for me, too," Gwyneth says. "A butterfly landed on the back of my hand. It opened its wings and circled around me. It was a sign from God."

A woman hands me a paper that says, "My Life Story As I See It, by

Mary Becker." ("You can put it in your book but only if you use my real name," she instructs me.)

"I write a weekly Newsletter here at Oasis. I AM Communications. I have no hearing. It all began with Alma, my domineering mother who always had to be Right and Jane an Older sister who got All the attention. Everything Alma or Jane said, I defied in WORDS. I let them know. I EXIST!"

Mary worked in public relations for the College of Nurses of Ontario. "If there was a legal situation involving a nurse – let's say the headline reads, 'Nurse Tilda May Have Accidentally Murdered a Patient' – I would check the records and prepare briefing sheets for the directors. I have always worked with words," her story concludes.

Gwyneth nudges the footstool to invite me over. I sit on it at her feet.

"I went through the water like Christ. I was brought up in the church, lived my life in the church. I am a Baptist, born in Wales, married a Canadian soldier in the war. I made my own wedding cake and can make Welsh rarebit, haggis, and more." She smiles and clasps her hands together. "God talks to me. To him I will go one day. I am His. I am not afraid to die. I know I'll be sitting at Jesus's feet."

There's a poke on my shoulder. "I'm Alton." A short, seemingly timid man boldly motions me to come to him next. "I'm the new kid on the block. I've been here only two years, but I know everyone. When the ambulance takes one of us away, none of us like it. One lady had to go to the hospital, but she came back. When another lady got short of breath, we helped her put on her shoes, got her purse, and called the ambulance. I had her key, so I did her dishes."

Alton looks over at Gwyneth, sitting in her throne chair, watching us and listening to our conversation. "Queen Gwyneth," he says, blowing her a kiss.

"I'm leaving this chair behind," Gwyneth tells me of the comfy chair she's sitting in. "I'm only using it now, until I am returned to the

Lord." She has a banana in her hand, holding it like an ice cream cone. Queen Gwyneth, ensconced in her throne, well cared for, at peace, with no regrets, only memories of a full life lived in accordance with her beliefs. She smiles at her banana, peels it slowly, takes a dainty bite, and looks up to give me a wink goodbye. "God bless," she says, reaching out to clasp my hand.

Ruth is the last to give her endorsement of the Oasis. "I love living here. It's not a nursing home and you get more help here than you would in a retirement home. We all know each other's business and check up on one another. We're family."

As I drive to my hotel, I think of Audrey – and her opposite. The opposite of Audrey McClenaghan is Joyce Vincent. A year or so ago, I saw a documentary called *Dreams of a Life* and Joyce's story has stayed with me ever since. Camera shots of the yellowing newspaper headlines told the story: "Woman Dead in London Bed-Sit for Three Years" and "Skeleton Found on Sofa with Telly Still On." Only thirty-eight years old when she was found dead in her one-room flat in London, England, Joyce had been full of life, accomplished, and beautiful. In a photograph she looks like a young Whitney Houston. At one time, there were people in Joyce's life – a former boyfriend, co-workers, sisters, other tenants in the building. Had she withdrawn from them or had they abandoned her? How does someone die – poof! – and no one notices for three years?

The cause of Joyce's death remains unknown, but foul play has been ruled out. She'd been living in subsidized housing, didn't drink or do drugs. When the apartment was finally opened, her skeletal remains, intact and upright, were found on the sofa. The TV was still on to the BBC news, an unopened Christmas present lay on the floor beside her, a pile of mail had built up inside the front door, there were dishes from her last meal in the sink, the window was open, curtains flapping in the breeze, insects and cobwebs had taken over, and there was a thick layer of dust everywhere. It's one of the saddest stories I've ever heard.

———

By the time I make it to my hotel it's ten o'clock, and I'm beat. Hungry, too. I'm tempted to indulge and order that room service I was fantasizing about, however, on VON's tab, I can't bring myself to do it. I'd feel like the Canadian member of Parliament who was outted for staying at a ritzy hotel and spending sixteen dollars of taxpayers' money on a glass of orange juice, and was forced to resign in shame. I pick up the phone and order extra-spicy chicken wings and a Coke. With my coat over my nightgown I go down in the elevator to the restaurant to pay for it myself and bring it back to my room. *Self*-service is always best.

1:00 A.M., NOTE TO SELF

No more chicken wings!

(At least, not after midnight.)

7

SMILE

SOBER-WASTED. That describes the state I'm in this morning. After a restless night, I woke up queasy, still recovering from my late-night wing fest. It's seven o'clock and somehow I've managed to drag myself to the local community centre where I'm now busting a move on the gymnasium floor with Gladys, Delphine, Millie, Harvey, and Werner. Twistin' and jiving, we're moving to the beat with Ken, our SMART instructor, who's not too hard on the eyes. For Seniors Maintaining Active Roles Together, you have to be fifty-five-plus to qualify. I'm not quite there yet, but they let me in.

"I hope I can keep up," I joke.

"Don't worry, dear, just go at your own pace," Millie says in all seriousness.

We grapevine and do-si-do to Harry Belafonte's "Day-O" and the Bee Gees' "Stayin' Alive." Last time I heard that song I was working in the ICU, caring for a patient whose condition was deteriorating. The song came on the bedside radio my patient's wife had put on earlier that morning. The unfortunate irony was that her husband was struggling to do that very thing. The wife and I glanced at each other, acknowledging the truth of those words. Come to think of it, "Stayin' Alive" is also the tune we play in our head while performing CPR on a patient during a cardiac arrest. The beat of that song's tempo helps us pace our chest compressions.

I'm in yoga pants and a plain black T-shirt. Wisely, I decided just before leaving my hotel room to change out of my colourful "No More War" T-shirt, emblazoned with a huge peace sign. I didn't think it would be welcomed here, in Trenton, a military town and home to the headquarters of Canada's largest air force base. Here, you see khaki camouflage and military personnel everywhere you go.

Trenton is also a down-home sort of place, with local eateries like Granny's Kitchen and Momma's Diner. A vintage sign says "Kentucky Fried Chicken," not KFC, the acronym now used, no doubt to mask the mention of grease. Downtown Trenton has one main drag, with businesses like Scrapbook and Smiles, a Dollarama, and a diner boasting the "Best Caesar Salad of the Season."

After exercise class it's time to visit the foot clinic.

Feet, it turns out, are a big deal. Who knew? In the ICU we don't pay attention to feet unless they're impressive: black with necrosis, red from inflammation, green with pus, or about to fall off for one reason or another. I've seen some gnarly feet in my day – mottled and dripping, scaly and lizard-like, even mummified, shrivelled, and flaky as parchment. Don't get me started.

Wally is Nurse Janet's first client. He settles into the chair, puts his feet up, and is pleased to have the attention of a "reporter" like me.

"If you've got a foot fetish, this is the place to be," says Wally, a jovial, burly, healthy-looking gentleman in his seventies, here for his six-month foot checkup. While Janet examines his feet, Wally doesn't waste a moment and launches straight into his life's story. "I'm a retired cop and I've been on a twenty-six-year vacation from liquor. I've taken a permanent holiday from the stuff." He makes abstinence sound delightful. "For years, my beat was downtown Toronto. I patrolled those mean streets for years and survived to tell the tale. Once I got in a brawl with an Asian prostitute who kicked me and knocked the cartilage out of my knee. She was all hopped up on drugs, along with another hooker – a black chick – and their Gino pimp."

What the relevance of the ethnic background of these characters is, I don't get a chance to ask, because Janet wants to tell me about her work and the standards maintained in this clinic. "We use sterile instruments that have been autoclaved. That's gold standard. Others may use antiseptic, but it doesn't kill everything."

"'Put your lawn mower up for sale,' my doc told me," interjects Wally. "If that's what a heart attack is, I'll have one every day. A twinge of indigestion, was all. Now, I take it easy."

Janet digs in between Wally's toes, gets under the nails. "How do you manage to wash your feet?" she asks him.

"I nailed a face cloth to a stick and use it to get down in between my toes," he says with a grin. Janet recommends a fungal spray, which will be easier for him to use.

"Wally has normal, healthy feet," she pronounces. "Beautiful feet."

"It must be from walking on sandy beaches. I'm a snowbird." Wally is one of those retired Canadians who escape to Florida for a certain number of winter days, careful not to overstay their sojourn and jeopardize their coveted health coverage.

Janet shows me her equipment. "We use heavy nippers. No grinding tools because they aerosolize any nail fungus that's present."

Discretely, I move my coffee cup out of the trajectory of any flying fungi.

Another client waiting for Janet's magic hands motions me over. "I want to tell my story, too. Don't forget about me. I don't want to get left out. And please use my real name – Fred Carson, by the way."

No concerns about "privacy" here, I see.

"It's Betty's turn," Janet tells him. "You're next, Fred."

"So pipe down, Fred, and take a number," Wally calls out from the sidelines.

Betty takes up her position in the feet seat, moving slowly and cautiously. She's a plump woman in her sixties who looks worried.

While Nurse Janet works on her feet, Betty talks to me. "Janet always tells me I have to be more careful, take better care of myself. I'm a diabetic and have almost no feeling in my feet. Once, Janet pulled out a pin that was stuck in my toe. I didn't even know it was there. Didn't feel a thing. Trimming my nails is impossible because I can't bend down."

(Now that I think of it, there was a memorable "foot" incident in the ICU. I can still hear the surgeon bellowing, "Will someone wash this woman's feet?" The patient's nurse informed him about the provenance of the deep grooves and dark striations in her patient's feet. "This woman is from India and has worked barefoot all her life in the rice fields. Her feet are not dirty." Not the least bit chastened, the surgeon stormed off.)

Nurse Janet remains focused on the foot at hand, Betty's.

"People think all we do is a leisurely pedicure, but professional foot care saves legs and is a lot cheaper than admitting them to a hospital for an amputation. Many elderly can't even reach their feet."

"It's quite a *feat*!" Wally quips from the peanut gallery.

(I guess he's staying to hang out, like in an old-school barber shop.)

"You can tell a lot about a person's health by examining their feet."

"Oh, the agony of *da-feat*."

(Guess who?)

"Once, I noted a client had foot drop and other neurological changes in just one of his feet," Janet recalls. "I was concerned, so I alerted his physician, and good thing I did because it turned out the man had a spinal tumour. He had surgery and is all right now."

"That's impressive detective work," I say.

"Make sure to use my real name. Wally Smitherman. I've got fungus on my left toe and my big toes are gouty. Tell the world. I don't give a hoot about privacy."

"I'm not sure your story will make the cut, Wally," I tease him. "My readers need more excitement than your healthy feet."

He looks bemused while I return my attention to Janet, who's talking radial pulses and pedal nerve innervations.

"Don't forget about me," he warns.

"How could we?" I assure him.

"I don't paint my nails. The reporter can quote me on that, also," he tells Janet.

"Duly noted, Wally," she says, then explains to me that clients pay a small fee for this service.

"Believe me, it's worth it," says Wally. "I wish I got paid for every bad guy I caught."

"We have a travelling clinic and do home visits for people who can't make it here."

"I'll miss you, Janet, when I'm in Florida."

Fred has been waiting patiently and, finally, it's his turn. He wants us to hear his whole story, not just about his feet.

"I did three tours in Germany during the war in the air force. I didn't want to sit in the slit tranches and couldn't swim, so the air force was for me."

"Veterans are covered to receive this service and it's free for those who can't afford to pay," Janet explains.

Fred uses his cane to slide his socks off. He can't reach his feet either.

Janet palpates his ankles. "Your ankles are swollen. Are you on a fluid pill?"

"Only a baby aspirin every second day."

Janet listens to his chest and hears bilateral crackles so she calls the doctor. Based on her findings, he orders a diuretic over the phone and a follow-up visit to his office tomorrow.

"Merry Christmas," Wally calls out as he gets ready to leave.

"It's only September," Betty says.

"Every day is a holiday when you're retired."

"I love feet," Janet says, going over to give Wally a goodbye hug. "And the people attached to them."

Deborah is a manager of the home care workers. She outlines their role, which is to prepare light meals, assist with personal care like bathing, showering, and dressing, and to help clients with their meds.

"They administer meds?" I ask. "Is that safe?"

"They are only allowed to cue them to take their meds, but if there's a concern or a change in the clients' health, they will call a nurse. Home care workers have different levels of education. It's difficult to find good ones. Let's face it: Who wants to work hard, deal with yucky things, cope with demanding, fussy people? Some are young and too good-hearted. If they see there's not enough food or clothes, they want to buy them, but they have to learn to set limits."

Deborah introduces me to Kendra Phillips, a home care worker who is on disability due to a work-related injury. After talking with Kendra for a few minutes, I get the feeling she's someone who struggles with those boundaries Deborah mentioned. In her twenties, with a short pixie cut and a sad face, she's been on long-term disability for the past few months. "I was helping a senior in the bathroom and he started to fall. We're not supposed to catch them, just guide them down to the floor, but he had cancer and was fighting a big battle, so I caught him. Immediately, I felt something tear in my shoulder."

"I can see you're in pain. What happened to the patient?"

"He passed away a few days later."

With her good arm, Kendra repositions the injured one, and winces from a sudden nerve spasm. "I feel guilty being off and not being there for my clients." Her eyes tear up. "I love my job but I have no idea when I'll be able to work again. My husband was an abusive control freak. I'm better off on my own, but I'm scared because if I can't work I have no idea how I'm going to support my two kids."

She doesn't move much or turn her neck. I'm an accurate detector of malingerers and embellishers, and I don't hear a *ding, ding, ding* around Kendra. Her pain is real and severe.

"VON has given me office work to do, like filing with my left hand, answering the phone." She stops to dab at her eyes. "Forgive me . . ."

"You're in pain." She nods, grateful that I recognize her suffering.

"I went back to work too soon and re-injured it. The thing is, I love my job. I love caring for seniors, especially ones with Alzheimer's or dementia. There's this one lady who has beautiful skin and it kills me that I'm not there to put her cream on her."

She tells me about another patient, one who had a big impact on her.

"She was a creature of habit and I learned those habits. At first she was difficult and cranky, but I didn't ask to be removed from the case. Eventually she told me, 'You are like one of my daughters.' But that made the daughters jealous. 'Mom's all yours,' they'd say to me. 'She only wants you anyway.' My client had these bad panic attacks and I was the only one who could talk her down. 'Take deep breaths,' I'd tell her. 'I'm here with you.' The day she had a stroke, I was there with her. She had told me many times she didn't want to be resuscitated in the event of something like that, but I didn't know how to make her comfortable. So, I called the ambulance. I told them she was a DNR and they listened to me. I kept telling her, 'stay with me, help is on the way.' When she died the daughters didn't let me come to the funeral. That hurt."

Kendra prides herself on her personalized care. "For one client, I used to always pick up her favourite treat – a walnut crunch doughnut and double-double coffee from Timmie's. I like to get to know their likes and dislikes. When I first meet a new client, I ask, 'What do you prefer I call you?' I took care of a Hélène who wanted her name pronounced the Quebecois way and got angry when anyone said Helen, the English way. People my age are used to speedy communication, so I make sure to slow down when I speak to seniors."

Next, I meet Mallory Freeburn and Leala Pardy, nurses who teach home care workers like Kendra. Mallory is mellow and sweet with frosted blond hair and Leala is tall and wears all-black; she has an edgy, rocker-girl vibe. They operate as a tag team and seem like they're long-time BFFs, but they've worked together for only a year. They speak in a rally of sound bytes and I sit back and listen to their verbal volleyball.

"You have to become what they need you to become," Leala starts off.

"But at the same time, encourage independence," Mallory joins in.

"It's challenging and not everyone is capable of it, but that's what's required."

"In the hospital, if you spend time with a patient, you'll get behind in your work and the other nurses will think you're lazy."

"Yeah," says Mallory. "I worked in a hospital and it was a bad experience. I'll never go back."

"I don't like hospitals, not one bit," Leala agrees. "The white rooms, white coats. It's stressful for staff, patients, family, and *sooo* political. They say you're part of a team, but as a nurse, I never felt it. In home care, you really are part of a team."

"Tell her what happened to you, Mal," Leala says. "Wait'll you hear this," she says to me.

"It was traumatic. I worked in a hospital dialysis unit and was under the microscope because I am a practical nurse and they were all registered nurses. They bullied me because they felt I might take their job and replace them. It even made the local newspaper. Eventually, I stood up to them. Now, I don't tolerate bullying in any way, shape, or form."

Leala smiles at Mallory and gets back to describing their job, teaching home care workers. "We teach them tact and diplomacy, because sometimes you go into a client's home and they're in a bad mood or uncooperative. They'll say they don't want a bath, but the smell tells you they need one," Leala says.

"Some ask to be taken to the liquor store or to buy lottery tickets or cigarettes," Mallory adds. "Some can be abusive, even request sexual favours. We teach the workers to be clear about what they are there to do."

"And *not* do," Leala adds, shooting Mallory a knowing look.

Mallory continues. "We go into some homes that should be condemned. You gag at the stink and feel revolted, but you have to put on your game face and not show your disgust. You have to put your judgements aside and be respectful because that's their home. It's their choice. Everyone has a right to live how they wish."

Leala describes a man who lives off the beaten path, off the grid entirely, in a 150-year-old old farmhouse. "Animals are running around, feral cats and dogs with missing legs and paws. Dog feces everywhere. There's a cage of birds with seeds and feathers all over its floor. The windows are dirty; you can't even see through them. The floor is so rickety, one nurse fell right through. So, I'm seeing this and all I can think is, OMG, OMG. This is the point where I have to compose myself and be a professional. You have to come to terms with the fact that you can't fix all the problems. You do what you can."

They continue on, completing and expanding on each idea, back and forth.

"There are definitely times when 'best practice' goes out the window. I remember one client who had a rash. The doctor prescribed cortisone cream, but the client was rubbing it with banana peels. It didn't get better, but that's what he wanted to do. Another guy kept his pills in his fishing tackle box, labelled 'Bill's Pills.' They were all mixed up in different bottles, some expired and without labels. He'd reach in and take whatever he grabbed a hold of. I wanted to get in there, go through all those medications and throw out the expired drugs, and the ones he didn't need, but he wouldn't let me. What can you do?" Leala raises her hands, palms up, to show her resignation to a fact that nurses often struggle with: there are some things we can't fix.

I'm embarrassed to think of how quick we are to label a patient uncooperative or non-compliant. Even "unmotivated" is a usual and equally damning label we use to describe patients who won't ambulate or engage in rehab. Once, we complained about our difficulty in getting an "unmotivated" patient to do more activity. But when his wife came in she said, "That's him. That's what he does at home – he lies on the couch and watches TV from morning to night. This is his usual level of activity." Who are we to try to get people to achieve *our* goals for them?

"Have you ever been in a situarion that felt dangerous?" I ask them.

"We always tell the home care workers, 'If your instinct tells you it's unsafe, don't go in, or get out immediately if you're already there. Never put yourself at risk.'" Mallory's answer reflects VON's policy, but Leala took matters into her own hands – literally.

"Once, I had to get a client to hand over his machete and let me confiscate it," she says casually, like it's nothing.

"Wow." *How cool is that?*

In Mallory's experience, it's more often the client who is the one in danger. "Once, we suspected a wife was abusing her husband. I was on the phone with her and she was speaking about him nicely, but when she put the phone down I heard her yelling and cursing at him. We went over to investigate. In another case, the husband left his wife alone in bed, lying in a wet diaper all day while he went off with his girlfriend. She was in bed with a broken hip that never healed properly."

Leala adds, "We ended up having to admit her to a long-term facility. There was no other way to keep her safe. We're the eyes and ears, right there on the scene. We take in everything. If something is wrong, we're the first to know about it."

In the afternoon, I meet Mae Quinn, a sprite, trim elder with a deeply lined face and an animated voice who's a proud VON volunteer. "I'm from Weyburn, Saskatchewan, and I've been a VON phone caller and friendly visitor for fifteen years."

We sit in the boardroom, but I wish I could see Mae in action, making her calls to folks at home.

"If I didn't have this outlet I'd be sitting at home, depressed. When you're alone, all you do is chew over your problems. *Oh, I'm alone, I'm so lonely.* If you volunteer, you help others fix their problems and end up fixing your own. I thought I was there to help them, but they're helping me." Mae's husband was in the military and they raised four kids together.

"Now, I call people who are alone and follow up if they don't answer. So many people have nobody in their lives. I visit shut-ins and chit-chat with them or play cards."

Mae misses her husband terribly. He died a year ago from pulmonary fibrosis caused by exposure to asbestos when he was a soldier during the war.

"Yes, he could have had surgery, but it was risky and he chose not to have it. He lasted one year. I wanted him to have the surgery, but my friend's husband spent his last year in the hospital, in constant pain. At least I have good memories, she keeps telling me. You didn't have to watch your husband suffer."

Mid-morning, I meet Don O'Neil, who gives me a hearty two-handed handshake. I accompany him on his rounds delivering meals cooked in the VON kitchen to people in need. He's a burly, handsome older man who takes anyone in his charge under his protective wing. He wears a dark-green soccer jersey with an Irish logo on it.

"My ancestors hale from the Emerald Isle," he says, proudly showing me his Claddagh ring. "If the heart points out, that means you're available. Heart facing inward means your heart is taken." (By the way, Don's faces out. Ladies, take note.)

"We have some very successful people here in Trenton. There are some people who make life better, others who make it worse." Don is a retired banker and now a "career volunteer-er." He says volunteering is not his hobby; he considers it his full-time job.

"I'm the Godfather of Trenton volunteers. I've been president of the Cancer Society, done sports charities. The military is very important here and many are VON volunteers. When one shows up at the door in uniform to deliver a meal, it's a real source of pride."

On the middle finger of his other hand, Don wears a Masonic ring, and just like every other Mason I've ever met (including my late father), he won't reveal the meaning of the secret symbol engraved on it. I wonder if these old-time clubs like Kiwanis, Knights of Columbus, and the Lions are still going strong? Do people these days still have those affiliations? Many young people I know go off to Africa or South America, or other developing or war-torn countries, to offer their services, but I often wonder if the needs right on our doorsteps, even though they're not as exotic or exciting, would attract them as well?

We pull into a driveway. "You can sit home and watch TV or get out and do something useful," Don says. "I don't like reality TV. I like *reality*. Yup, as a volunteer, I get a 100 per cent increase in my wage every year." He shoots me a wink.

In this house we meet Jerry, who was a golf pro until he had a stroke last year. He now uses a wheelchair and depends entirely on these delivered meals for his nutrition. Don is bringing him a ham sandwich for lunch and beef stew over rice for dinner. On the front door a sign says "No smoking, oxygen in use," yet the house reeks of smoke and Jerry's coughing a wet, bronchial cough.

"We're not here to judge," Don reminds me on the down low, as we're leaving.

Nancy's face lights up when she sees us on the doorstep with her meal. In her arms she cradles a chocolate poodle who probably weighs more than she does. He's definitely better nourished. With her teeny-tiny stick legs and arms, I wonder if Nancy is even sixty pounds. Her hands shake and she's unsteady on her feet. There is no way she could survive without these meals. She'd be admitted to a hospital with the diagnosis "failure to thrive," and be put on intravenous hydration and tube feedings. I wonder what's in her refrigerator right now. The meals Don brings are keeping Nancy alive.

"For some folks, we're their only human contact." Don and I are back in the car, on the way to the next delivery. "Well, I'm supposed to be retired, but I'm so busy, I think I'll go back to work to get a rest. Volunteering is something I do for myself. Abraham Lincoln said, 'When I do good, I feel good. When I do bad, I feel bad.'"

I'm still thinking about Nancy. I wonder if Don is too because he says, "If we see something not right we report it to the office and they come over to check." He pulls into the parking lot of a closed-down bar with dusty windows. Don is about to deliver a meal to a tenant in the seedy rooming house above the bar. "Stay in the car for this one," he says protectively. When he comes back down, he's sad. "I've seen that lady all around town with a child in tow. Bad teeth, ragged clothes. Can't tell if it's a girl or a boy. It reeked of marijuana up there. Maybe something worse than marijuana."

We drive on. "My wife would have benefitted from some of that. Medicinal marijuana, I mean." He gives me a sideways glance to check if I disapprove, which I don't. "She was dying of cancer, but her doctor wouldn't prescribe it."

We stop to deliver a meal to a man who's more interested in showing me the roses he planted in his garden in memory of his wife (of the same name) than the food delivery.

"There's lots of lonely people out here," Don tells me back in the car. "One lady would push her lifeline just to get the firefighters and police to come. But first, she'd put on lipstick and a spray of perfume." Don believes that people don't know how much fun it is to help others. "The best reason to do it is for yourself. Sure, there's the odd grumpy one, but if you look at their circumstances you can see why they might be like that."

What a pleasure it would be to have Don deliver me a warm, cooked meal in an insulated puffy bag, but I'm sure I don't qualify. Spending time with Don reminds me of how members of a close community can help each other. When my sons were little, we lived in a neighbourhood where I knew most of the people on the street, and the Di Tosto family were the best neighbours anyone could ever have. Time and again we counted on them and they always came through. We had keys to each other's houses and once, while we were on a family vacation, we called them to check if we'd left the stove on. (We hadn't.) They taught us how to put on our five-year-old's hockey gear his first time on the ice and how to take care of our shrubs and bushes (we are hopeless gardeners). I found ways to give back. They called upon me to give their teenage son injections he needed. In fact, I became known as the neighbourhood nurse to many on the street. I loved that role, being consulted by one neighbour over whether or not to take his kid's sprained ankle to the ER, doing a lice check, and even helping care for someone's father when he was recovering from a stroke. Unfortunately, we moved and our new 'hood isn't nearly as friendly. I often think I'd like to move back there.

SMILE – Seniors Managing Independent Life Easily – is a program to help keep seniors at home for as long as possible and out of long-term care facilities. They offer help with laundry, shopping, cooking, housekeeping, chores, and errands. I meet two recipients of this program – Edith, a seventy-year-old woman with a child-like, inno-cent smile who sits on the couch with Patrick, her husband and full-time caregiver. He says he's reconciled to his role, but I sense weariness in his tired eyes and downcast expression.

Edith has had to learn to walk and talk again after a brain aneurysm last year. A home care worker comes every day to help her bathe and get dressed, and to give Patrick a break.

"That's my time to get groceries, run errands, but sometimes all I do is sit in a bar and read the newspaper. Even if I do nothing, it's good to get out of the house. I can't leave her alone for even a moment. She gets confused about where she is and panics. Sometimes, she keeps going to the bathroom because she forgets she just went."

"You have a nice husband," I say to Edith.

"Yes, I do," she says excitedly, but then looks at Patrick's mournful face. "I used to be a good wife, but I'm no good to him anymore."

"You're still good," he tells her, leaning over to pat her hand.

"Poor honey," Edith says, her mood abruptly changing from cheer-ful to sad. "You don't have fun anymore, do you? I've ruined his life," she tells me, and starts to cry.

Patrick puts his arm around her. "No, dear, it's fine."

One thing that makes caring for Edith very difficult for Patrick is his own health problems – migraines, arthritis, and early signs of Parkinson's disease.

"At times, it all falls apart, but somehow, we muddle through," he says.

"Patrick was an engineer, and was offered a job in Africa. He loves adventure and wanted to go but I didn't," Edith says.

"I'd forgotten all about that," he says softly.

Clearly, she's got the long-term memory and he, the short. Together, they're a team. The highlight of each month is dinner at the Lion's Club held at the church.

"This isn't how I thought we'd live out our golden years." Patrick's voice trails off as he looks out the window.

My last stop of the day is a community centre where I sit at an oval-shaped table with seniors who have suffered brain injuries or cognitive deterioration and have come here for a day of conversation, light exercise, games, and crafts. The walls are decorated with cheap and cheerful displays of their artwork—collages, drawings, and paintings. In some of the portraits, faces are fragmented and distorted—a reflection of the way they see these images.

A man with an English accent starts up a conversation with me in halting, slow speech. "I'm Herman, originally from Cornwall, England."

"What do you like about coming here?" I ask.

"The company," he says, but seems to be thinking about something else he wants to tell me about himself. "I'm the one who laid out the first cloverleaf on a highway in Canada."

"You designed it?"

"No, I laid it out."

"So, you built it?"

"No, I laid it out. I'm a surveyor."

Remind me, please. Who's the cognitively impaired one here?

Charlotte, the director of the adult day program, shows me wooden nickels they use for a game. "Yes, we're gambling, but *shhhhh*. Don't tell anyone."

Around the table, one by one, each person introduces themselves. When Bart says his name, he inexplicably bursts into tears. Charlotte leans over to comfort him.

Sally, a vivacious woman, speaks next. "I'm from Scotland. A plain, no-nonsense lass am I."

"No kidding." Freda cuts her off. "We know you're from Scotland. Your accent?"

"Aye, this lassie loves to be chased by lads in kilts," Sally agrees.

Maurice raises his finger, requesting a turn to speak. "I was a supply technician in England during the War. Double-U, Double-U Two."

"Oh, he's been around," Freda pipes up. "Now, back to me. It was my turn. I've been blind since I was ten. I was born with cataracts on the lenses of my eyes. Now they can fix a problem like that. Even when I had three babies in diapers, I cooked and cleaned. I can knit anything that pops to mind. I sewed my girls' clothes on a sewing machine. Dresses with ruching, puffed sleeves, zippers . . ."

Ouch. "How did you keep your fingers out of the way of the needle?"

"I felt my way along. I had a good sense of where the needle was. My mother taught me, but she died when I was six. My father made axe handles, got a few dollars for each one."

This library of human books has it all: history, romance, comedy, tragedy.

Later, back at the VON office, staff are buzzing with excitement. Up until now, it's been a secret, but it's time to make an announcement: Judith Shamian will be starring in an episode of the reality TV show *Undercover Boss*. She had told me about posing as an entry-level employee, working in a disguise of glasses, a frumpy wig, a dowdy pink sweater, and scuffed running shoes. She looked completely different than her polished chic style and must have played the part so well that no one recognized her. The promo states:

As baby boomers age, there's increased demand on homecare services. VON cares for people in their own homes. Once unique, now rival companies compete for the business. Judith Shamian worries this Canadian institution will be consigned to the history books. She will be in disguise so she can see for herself what's really going on in the front lines.

Anticipation is in the air.

8

IT'S A BEAUTIFUL DAY IN THE HOSPITAL

I'VE BEEN ON THIS ASSIGNMENT for two months and so far haven't faced any emergencies or saved any lives, but even *sans* adrenaline rush, I'm having a great time. It's fun being on the road, meeting interesting people, and learning new things. Everyone is so upbeat and positive. Indeed, the world outside the hospital is pleasant. Who knew? But I keep having an uneasy feeling . . . that what they're showing me is maybe *too* pleasant?

Something is wrong with this picture. There's a dark side. The earworm "It's a Beautiful Day in the Neighbourhood" plays in my head, more saccharine than sweet. Yes, there's Audrey, doted upon by friends and caregivers; Ken and Pat coping brilliantly with home dialysis; stalwart Patrick, tenderly caring for Edith – but are they the norm or the exception?

I happen to know it's not all rainbows and blue skies out there. I've read about elder abuse, burnt-out caregivers, a shortage of home care services and long-term facility beds. Given all of that, why is VON showing me only the sunny side, the success stories?

Fortunately, I have a few sources to get the inside scoop. Magda, a former ICU nurse, is now a geriatric emergency manager (GEM). She's

agreed to allow me to visit her where she works, in the ER of a big downtown medical centre. (It's a "bones and groans," she'd said, meaning a
general hospital, and "strictly BBCSs" – bumps, bruises, cuts, and
scrapes. "No trauma or anything exciting like that, Tilda, if that's what
you're looking for.") But she'll only meet with me surreptitiously, on a
quiet, Sunday morning when no administrators are around. She asks
me not to use her real name and looks uneasy about talking with me.
I've often wondered why nurses are hesitant to speak up. Why are they
fearful? Nurses have so much to say but often stay silent. Judith was
right about that. Despite her initial hesitation, it doesn't take Magda
long to show her true feelings – which are frustration and outrage. In
fact, when I start by asking her about her GEM training, straight out of
the gate she explodes with vehemence.

"The best training would be at a debt collection agency," Magda
says. "You have to nag people, make them feel guilty that they came to
the hospital. We're supposed to be a brick wall, not a sieve, and not
admit anyone. It's not a *directive* but that's the message management
gives us." Magda wears a crisp white lab coat over casual clothes, cor-
duroy pants and a T-shirt. A stethoscope hangs out of one pocket and
the pocket on the other side sags from the weight of her phone, a reflex
hammer, and her wallet. Her appearance is professional, but her tousled bright red hair and flushed cheeks make her seem like she's got
skin in the game, like an indignant family member, complaining about
the substandard care her own parents are receiving.

"The emergency department is the worst place for an elderly person
but they come here because they have nowhere else to go, and our job
is to send them back home," she says as we sit at the nursing station to
review the list of patients currently in the ER. Among others, there's a
fifty-year-old homeless man with a fever, a child with a stomach ache,
a teenager who is threatening to jump off a bridge, a distraught fifty-
six-year-old woman who hasn't slept for three nights in a row, an
eighty-eight-year-old man who had a "neurological episode," and a
seventy-year-old woman with pains in her arm, plus a few more.

They've all been triaged, with top priority for a "one," which is stroke, head trauma, hemorrhage, or possible heart attack, all the way down to the "fives," who are the walking wounded.

"They're like, 'Really? Why are you here?'" as Magda puts it. "Some of these people make me wonder if they'd have come here at all if they had someone to care for them at home." She nods over at a wild-eyed person who looks like he lives on the street. "Or, if they had a home, which is what our febrile 'urban outdoorsman' needs." The man she's referring to is sitting in a row of chairs inside the treatment area along with ten other worried-looking people, none of whom appear, at least outwardly, to be experiencing an emergency.

"They're the 'chair people,'" Magda says, "the 'breakfast club.' They've passed triage, they're making progress, so it lessens their stress."

Since Magda's specialty is geriatrics, she zeroes in on the "crinklies and wrinklies" whose only crime is "TMB – too many birthdays."

(Please note: hospital slang can be deceiving. The assumption is that people who use these crude short-forms are callous and unfeeling. Paradoxically, it's often the opposite. I know wonderful, caring nurses and doctors who speak this way, and terrible ones who never do. I'll take the wisecracking nurse who actually cares over the sweet-talker who's only keeping up a pretense. As for Magda, despite her jokey talk, I feel how deeply she cares.)

Magda charges forth to our first patient. "We'll start with the 'neurological episode.' Probably a stroke or AGI – 'acute gravity incident.' You know, FDGB – fall down go boom. Falls are the most common reason an elder comes to the ER."

We wend our way though the noisy, crowded treatment area where patients are either waiting in individual private rooms or lying in the hallways on gurneys around the nursing station. One of these is Magda's patient, a seventy-year-old man who's unwashed, unshaven, and barefoot, wearing only a flimsy hospital gown. He'd been on his way to the kitchen without his walker and fell over his cat. He got to the phone and called 911. "I didn't want to call the kids and bother them on the weekend." His only complaint is feeling "weak and dizzy."

"'Weak and dizzy' – that's what they all say," Magda says to me. "We have to ask a lot of questions, tease it out, figure out the puzzle." Magda does that and examines him at the same time. She finds good range of motion, and some sensitive areas and bruises on his back and legs. After ruling out injury from the fall, she advises him to use a walker, get rid of scatter rugs, and put bars in the shower. Magda admits her advice may or may not be followed.

"He's on the edge. If I had the time, I'd do a cognitive assessment and delve into how he's been managing since his wife died. There are lots of red flags that need follow-up, but that's not part of my job. We'll send out a home care nurse to assess the situation, but for now, he'll go back home, but will probably come back at some point. His diagnosis? ALC."

"Alternate level of care?"

"No. À la casa. Remember, T 'n' T is our mantra."

"What? Tea and toast?" It's the known fallback meal of elders living alone.

"No, Treat and Turf, as brutal as it sounds. Remember, 'brick wall,' not 'sieve.' I'll get a bad rep if I admit too many. Okay, let's go see the woman with the pain in her arm."

"I took my nitro, it didn't help." A well-groomed, bejewelled lady in white tennis shoes lies on the stretcher, her purse clutched to her side. Magda does an ECG and asks her about her pain, but the woman's answer reflects another agenda. "My rent went up by thirty-four dollars, but I still have my mind, thank God. My husband will have a word with the landlord." Magda orders blood work, asks more questions, then we step aside for her to fill me in. "She's a multi-millionaire widow who's a frequent flyer. She comes here every weekend on her housekeeper's day off. We can't admit her – normal vitals, an unremarkable ECG, and mild confusion won't cut it – but it's not safe for her to go home. Diagnosis? NPTG – no place to go." Magda's only recourse is to call a niece who agrees to come get her, but only later this evening.

The ER — not only a walk-in clinic and a hotel, but now an adult day care.

Magda knows the next patient, too, an eighty-six-year old woman with frontal lobe dementia. "The brain shrinks to the size of a walnut, then a grape," Magda explains. The husband brings her in when she doesn't take her meds and gets aggressive. This morning he woke up to her hitting and kicking him and threatening to stab him.

"She didn't mean it," he excuses her. "It's not her. She's really very sweet."

Magda tells me that home care case managers (aka "care coordinators," plus other titles) — the professionals who go into clients' homes to assess what services are needed — have visited her at home, but each time she rallies and acts somewhat normal. They have urged the husband to put her in a nursing home for his own safety, but he can't bring himself to do it. Besides, she would need a locked ward that can handle violent patients, and there's a shortage of those beds.

Magda is more worried about the husband than the wife. From the nursing station, we observe him standing at her side. He's exhausted and frightened, hunched over, his eyes downward, looking ashamed, like all victims of abuse. Despite the danger to him, Magda has no choice but to send them home.

"At least he got a few hours of respite here with us," she says wearily. *The ER is now a patient lock-down, a caregiver sanctuary.*

"Let's hope we don't read that she murdered him in tomorrow's newspaper," Magda mutters.

Next!

Nurses often feel stressed, but I'm not stressed. I'm *distressed*. In thirty years as a nurse, I've seen many shocking things, but never anything as disturbing as this, never as many unsafe situations, elders not getting the care or treatment they need. It's shocking and frightening, too — because we'll all be there ourselves, one day — or someone we love will be.

"We pray for a urinary tract infection or a fracture so we have a reason to admit them for 'crisis placement,' just to give the family a breather. But

if we admit them they'll become bed blockers, waiting for placement –
that phrase makes them sound like a piece of furniture, doesn't it?"
Magda pauses briefly to come up for air, then dives back down to continue her rant. "For seniors, a hospitalization is a huge setback. Every
day in bed, they lose 5 per cent of muscle mass and thus mobility."

Yet, once discharged home, alarming new problems ensue. One in
six patients is readmitted to hospital within ten days of discharge
home; one in five elderly patients is readmitted within ten days. Most
of these readmissions would not have been necessary if there had
been proper follow-up care. Unbelievably, the cost of readmission to
hospital for these avoidable problems amounts to a $1.8 billion drain
on the health care system.

"One lady was discharged home even though she wasn't able to
ambulate to the bathroom and she had no one to buy a commode for
her. 'Sure, we'll save your life, but we can't get you a potty.' As for
physiotherapy after a hip replacement or speech therapy after a stroke,
you only get three visits. Yet walking and talking make all the difference in a person's quality of life, wouldn't you agree? In the hospital,
patients get everything they need, but next to nothing at home. It's
basically YOYO – you're on your own. It's no wonder that a few days
later they *bounce back atcha* here in the ER."

Magda explains what I've known for a long time. Patients are sicker
than ever and hospital stays are shorter than ever. People are sent
home too soon, in a fragile condition, and have to cope with oxygen,
medications, IVs, drains, and dressings in a debilitated condition. It's
no wonder they develop complications and need readmission. It's easy
to see why caregivers feel overwhelmed and can't cope. "But why do
the surgery in the first place if patients can't recover at home properly?" Magda asks.

Yet, in all fairness, Magda acknowledges that some people's expectations are out of line. "They expect five-star service. One lady complained that her 'demands aren't being met,' and asked for 'someone
to come over to cut up my carrots.' An argument could be made that a

mani and a pedi are good for mental health, but should the government cover that, too? Where do we draw the line on services we can
offer? Canadians are not used to paying for health care, but we can't
provide everything to everyone all the time. Choices have to be made."

I'm getting the picture: there's a shortage of long-term care beds.
Home is where people want to be, but it's not always the safest place.
Family caregivers struggle to give care, but get pushed to the brink, which
can lead to abuse or neglect. Magda knows of families who keep a parent
at home just so they won't lose the parent's pension income, which would
go to the nursing home. She tells me about "granny-dumping." "One
grown-up daughter abandoned her elderly mother on the ER doorstep,
saying she simply couldn't cope with her anymore. Neighbours came to
pick her up, but she wandered off and was found in the basement of the
apartment building in a nightgown, babbling incoherently."

Magda asks if I want to see more, but no, I've seen enough. For
today, anyway. But just as I'm about to leave it all behind me, I notice a
security guard escorting two homeless women to the door. A nurse
follows close behind, telling them gently, "It's just that you come here
all the time." They look at her with imploring eyes. "I'm sorry but
there's nothing we can do for you."

I don't blame her. What, really, *can* she offer them?

For years my friend Annie has been telling me about her work. She's a
public health nurse who counsels "at-risk" mothers living in "high-
risk neighbourhoods." When describing what she does, she mentions
terms I'm unfamiliar with, such as "fostering maternal attachment"
and the "social determinants of health." I ask her to explain.

"It's about helping the baby and mother connect to each other,"
Annie says. "It's about the effect of poverty, diet, unemployment, education, and homelessness, on people's health."

Apparently, "high-risk" doesn't mean hypertension, diabetes,
high cholesterol, and lifestyle choices, which is how we define it in the
hospital. Out here, "high-risk" means poverty, drugs, crime, new

immigrants, or refugees fleeing disaster zones or oppressive regimes. I ask if I can visit her at work. I need to see it – no, experience it, first-hand – to understand it. But Annie deals with sensitive, sometimes politically charged situations. There would be scads of red tape and administrative hoops to get through for me to be allowed to visit. It would too long to arrange. I'm disappointed, but let it go.

The other ongoing annoyance is that Judith has not returned my calls or emails. (Where in the world is she? It's not "Where's Waldo?" but "Where's Judith?" Mogadishu? Bukhet? Hong Kong? You'd need a GPS to keep up with her. No wonder she jokes that, asked where she lives, she answers "Air Canada.") But suddenly, the reason for her silence dawns on me. September is the time of year for the High Holy Days. First, there's Rosh Hashanah, the Jewish New Year; then Yom Kippur, the Day of Atonement; Sukkot, the Festival of Thanksgiving; and Simchat Torah, a celebration of the Torah. Judith is busy with family celebrations and synagogue attendance and I likely won't hear from her for a few more weeks.

At least there's Audrey. Since returning home from Trenton last week, I've received three letters from her – toadstools, autumn leaves, black cats, and orange pumpkins on these ones – including clippings of articles on health care, about new books she thinks I'd like, or about the Kemptville Panthers junior hockey team, for my sons. There are questions, too, which I answer in my reply, and then a request. But first, she presents her latest vital signs.

October 15, 2012 0845 hours
Sugar 13.7
B.P. 119/61
Heart 63
Stable condition

Why do nurses wear such big watches?
Younger ones use their smartphones to tell time.

Is it better for your heart to sleep on your right side or your left?
It doesn't matter. Whichever side is more comfortable for you.

Was the SARS outbreak your worst nursing experience?
It was definitely scary, but I felt proud to be a front-line nurse at
*   that time.*

Does VON stand for "Very Outstanding Nurses"?
No, but I will pass on your suggestion.

My dear Nurse Tilda,
Promise me you will come to my 8oth birthday bash. It will be on
February 6th, if I make it till then. It would be a dream come true
to have you there. Please don't let me down.

It's October. Four months away. I write back to tell her to stay alive
and I'll try to be there.

9

SHWARMA AND HUMMUS AT DR. LAFFA

NEWS FLASHES FROM THE ICU ... beep, beep, beep ... wait for it ...
Rita got a baby! (A six-month-old girl she adopted from China.)

Joni is engaged! (Boy, that was fast. Didn't she just meet the guy a
month ago?)

Sadly, Malcolm's mother died. (He took care of her at home these
past few months.)

I've been keeping up with my ICU peeps on Facebook, but you can't
hug or congratulate or console in the virtual world like you can in the
real one, so I'm here in person to coo over baby pics with Rita, admire
the sparkle on Joni's hand ("fairy dust," she calls it), and comfort
Malcolm – plus work a twelve-hour day shift in the ICU. That niggling
apprehension I always get whenever I've been away from the ICU, the
worry that I've lost my touch, disappears within minutes as my confidence returns and I'm back in the zone, capably caring for a patient
who is three days post-op abdominal surgery for a bowel obstruction
and still intubated and heavily sedated.

"Welcome back," they all exclaim when I arrive at the nursing station at the beginning of a day shift. "Where've you been?"

"Are you broke? Is that why you're back?"

"Perhaps a bad case of writer's block? Need some new material?"

No, none of the above. I love it here, I keep telling them. This is home. I've been travelling, doing some research. A few more weeks, then I'll be back at work as usual.

"What's it like?" they all ask (silently smug, I'm sure, ready with their *I told you so's*).

"Interesting," I say mysteriously, leaving it at that. *Fascinating*, in fact, but they wouldn't have believed me (nor would I have, if I hadn't experienced it myself). Nor could I have explained why. I'm still figuring it out. But for today, it's great to be back in my stomping grounds with old friends. After all, laughing and eating lunch together with your pals is another thing you can't do in cyberspace, isn't it? After all, *life is with people*.

Life Is with People was the title of a treasured book in my father's library. It was about the Polish *shtetl* at the turn of the century, and the tight communities of Jews whose daily lives were interconnected through celebrations, losses, and everyday activities. My father loved that book, and I still have his copy with his handwritten notes in the margins and entire paragraphs highlighted. Whenever I spent too much time hiding indoors during my shy, reclusive childhood or my loner teenager years, my father would point to that book on the shelf. "Don't shut yourself away," he'd say, paraphrasing from the Talmud, the book of rabbinic commentary on the Torah. "Life is with people."

But I haven't closed myself off from the disturbing scenes I witnessed the other day with Magda. None of it was a complete surprise to me, but to see it up-close-and-personal brought it home. For some time now, it's been hard to miss the screaming headlines in the *Toronto Star*: "Seniors in Crisis, Begging for Care," "Family Caregivers Overwhelmed," and "Home Care Is Broken." Like everyone else, I've known about this crisis (predicted to only get worse with our aging, chronically ill population), but only vaguely and from a distance. The whole subject has been a bit like being aware of a genre of music that you chose to avoid, thinking you won't like it. *That kind of music is not my taste,* you tell yourself. Yet, when you decide to open yourself up to it, you surprise yourself by getting into it. Or maybe it's like learning a word for a concept that had previously been a formless, emerging awareness in your brain – highbrow words like *inchoate* or *ubiquitous*, let's say. Suddenly, that word pops up everywhere you go. Is it something new, or was it always there but you weren't attuned to it?

The crisis of care of our growing senior population is all over the zeitgeist: the "ticking time bombs," "the Grey Tsunami," "Baby Boomerangst." In my own online research, I've read articles that Judith has written on this subject and she has a different take. She believes that seniors are being demonized, blamed for the out-of-control spending in health care. "That's a myth," she says, calling it "senior bashing" and "ageism" and writes, "One would think that seniors are going to singlehandedly destroy the world as we know it – or, at least, bankrupt the healthcare system." She argues that caring for our aging population is only a modest health care cost driver, accounting for a mere 1 per cent increase in health care spending; that can't explain skyrocketing health care costs. Spending on seniors isn't growing at a faster rate than spending for the population at large. Judith argues that health care costs are rising due to expectations from the public to receive more and more services – including new drugs, expensive hospital care, and the latest technological advances – and especially due to the relatively new financial burden created by the increase in chronic illnesses.

As soon as the Jewish holidays were over, I finally snagged a meeting with Judith, again in her home, this time on a Sunday afternoon. I was hoping to talk with her about these serious issues. So, we're back in her front living room, by a large window that looks onto a quiet street, sitting side by side in the comfortable chairs. I suppressed a little giggle, imagining us as two pundits sitting on a panel, squaring off on a current events TV show like *Agenda* or *Meet the Press*. The little table between us was once again stacked with books and journals, different ones than on my last visit. Sneaking a peek while she took a phone call, I saw an issue of the *Harvard Business Review*, a biography of Barbra Streisand, and, again, the heavy Hebrew bible with the blue silk ribbon bookmark trailing out resting on top of the pile.

There's something reassuring, even appealing – at least to me – about a leader keeping a religious book so close at hand. Even though I'm not a believer, I like that she is. If taken to heart, the moral teachings and words of wisdom could keep a leader true to good values.

Judith turned off her phone, placed it on the table, and gave me her full attention. Wasting no time, I launched into my rant about the crisis in home care, its disorganization and inadequacy, the neglect of seniors, the shortage of long-term beds, the overwhelmed caregivers.

At first, Judith listened closely, but when I paused, she spoke.

"It is painful to witness human suffering." She looked out the window onto the quiet street for a few moments. "Let's go out for a bite to eat," she said unexpectedly.

Deflated, I wondered if she'd heard me. (I am also beginning to wonder if Judith cooks. On *Undercover Boss*, disguised as a home care worker, she acted inept, bumbling around in the client's kitchen. She didn't even know how to make toast. Was she playing a role, or was that really her? I don't exactly smell any chicken soup with matzah balls simmering on the stove or chocolate chip cookies baking in the oven when I visit her home.) We got into my car and drove to nearby Dr. Laffa, a kosher middle-eastern "meat" restaurant, a designation that differentiates it from a "dairy" restaurant. According to the rules of keeping kosher, meat and dairy products are not to come in contact with one another.

As we waited to be served, I got back to my concerns.

I told her about visiting Magda in the hospital and the problems I witnessed there – seniors jamming up the ER, sent home to unsafe situations, "crisis placement," "caregiver fatigue," readmissions after hospitalization, et cetera (lots of et ceteras).

Suddenly, I realized that, again, Judith was not listening to me. Her mind was far away. I was getting exasperated. I started to think about how I might weasel my way out of this frustrating assignment,

when suddenly, it dawned on me. Judith is working on these problems from a completely different angle. In fact, she knows them so
well, and is so deeply concerned about them, that she's chosen to
focus on their solutions. I'm in the past, still weaning myself off old
ways of thinking, trying to grasp new ones; she's fully engaged in
bringing about that old, long-predicted titanic paradigm shift that
has been talked about for so long – turning the focus to wellness,
primary care, and home care.

*I always feel a few steps behind her, straining to keep up with her
fast mind and boundless energy. I can almost feel the force field of her
brain, the heat of her bristling intelligence, pulsing like a living thing
around her.*

"Our health care system does not need more money," she said. "It
requires something more difficult – imagination and creative vision,
attention to basic human needs, and courage. Courage is needed to do
things differently and lead the way."

Sheepishly, I put aside the folder of articles I'd clipped from newspapers to prove my points. Luckily, the food arrived and I was instantly
distracted by the luscious, flaky laffa bread, slightly smoky from the
wood-burning oven, and the rich, creamy, lemony hummus, crispy
falafel balls, and smoky eggplant salad. I tried to pay attention to what
Judith was saying.

"From your travels, you are just beginning to scratch the surface of
the problems, the inequities, the unmet needs, the results of a system
overly focused on sickness and hospital care. Spending more on hospitals will not make us healthier. Health has little to do with hospitals
or medical intervention. At VON, we say, 'Health Starts at Home,' but
many people do not even have a home."

She gave me a few moments to take all that in while she served me – a
hefty portion of stewed mushrooms and spicy grilled chicken – then
herself. "People are living longer, but with more chronic illnesses. But
what if a person with diabetes receives good primary care? They'd be
less likely to later need dialysis, amputation, or hospitalization."

In the ICU I have cared for many people with diabetes and its complications; they are at the end stage of these problems. What Judith
was describing was the other end of the spectrum — preventing these
problems altogether.

I must have looked as discouraged as I felt because she threw me a
bone. "We have to roll up our sleeves and get to work, especially when
these problems are all fixable."

After we finished eating, we sat back. Judith was in a mood to
reminisce.

"My life has been about building relationships, connecting with
people. I have colleagues and friends around the world." Of all her many
achievements, that seemed to be the one of which she's most proud. By
now, I know her bio pretty well. Born in Hungary, a child of Holocaust
survivors who escaped to Israel; English is her third language. She studied
nursing in Jerusalem, married, came to Canada at twenty-five, worked as
a nurse at the Jewish General in Montreal, got a master's degree, then a
Ph.D., became Chief Nurse of Canada, then president of the Canadian
Nurses' Association, and is now running for president of the International
Council of Nurses (ICN), the largest worldwide organization of nurses.

She is passionate about our socialized health care system. She told
me about her time in Ottawa at the Office of Nursing Policy. "My small
apartment there had a view of the flag on the top of the Peace Tower. It
served as a daily reminder of my commitment to do everything I can
to advocate for sustaining our health care system for the future."

On the personal side, I asked her about any mentors she'd had
along the way. Her first was her director of nursing, a woman named
Mary Barrett.

"Mary was prim and proper," Judith said. "A real lady, with every hair
in place. There I was, a new nurse, an immigrant straight off the boat, a
staff nurse with little experience who could barely speak English. She
must have seen something in me because she made me a manager. Years
later, I asked her why she hired me. 'I needed a "troublemaker,"' she
said, 'someone to stir the pot, and I knew that was you.'"

The reason I asked her about mentors is because the topic has been on my mind a lot lately. I receive many emails from young nurses who say they want to find a mentor but have had no luck; the nurses they encounter are either too busy or too burnt-out to offer them any guidance. Just the week before, I had received this email.

Dear Nurse Tilda,
I recently graduated from university and am now starting out on my nursing career. I don't have a job yet, but I'm looking for a mentor. How do I find one? Do you know anyone willing to mentor me? Can you help me?
Sincerely, New Nurse

Apparently, mentors are in short supply. My advice? Keep on the lookout; they are out there, but know what you're getting into. A mentor doesn't make life easier; a good mentor will raise the bar and challenge you. The mentor's job is not to hold your hand or stroke your back, but to light a fire under you and kick your ass. Take it from me – Beware, *and be wary*, of the mentor. Life is definitely easier without one. Be honest with yourself: if it's encouragement you are looking for – and everyone needs some of that when starting out – find a cheerleader, a life coach, a good friend (or a bad therapist).

Judith repositioned her chair sideways, so she was sitting parallel to the table and pushed her glasses up to the top of her head. As she did, I noticed her beautifully manicured hands, a tiny daisy painted on each pinky finger. *This babe has a fun side – I hope I can get to know it.* Judith put her palms together and gazed out, beyond the other diners and the waiters carrying plates of food in this busy restaurant. "Mine is a Cinderella story. Imagine, a new Canadian like me running this great organization that's so much a part of our history. But it makes sense. VON is a complete expression of my personal values. If you want to see *chesed* and *tzedek*, they live at VON." She didn't translate for me; she trusted I knew these Hebrew words meaning "loving-kindness" and "justice."

"The most important thing is to be true to who you are and to your own values. I am not afraid to be a Jew in the world. As a Jew and as a nurse, I have an obligation to pursue *g'milut chasidim* – social justice. For me, being a Jew is inseparable from being a nurse, from being a CEO, from being a Canadian, from being a global citizen, from being a grandmother. All of these things encompass who I am."

She confided that her bid to become president of ICN has become a demanding and time-consuming campaign. She must travel constantly and work hard to become intimately familiar with the health care issues in each of the 135 countries that ICN represents. I would have thought she'd be a shoo-in, but apparently, the competition is fierce. "Taiwan has a very strong candidate," she says, "and Colombia, too."

Whatever it is that Judith does in the upper echelons of the United Nations and the World Health Organization remains invisible to me. It strains my imagination, so I do what I always do when I'm feeling out of my depth: I make a joke.

"Just think, if you become the ICN president, you'd be Nurse of the Universe," I teased her, not sure how she'd take it. "Hey," I forged on bravely, "that's even better than Miss Universe 'cause there's no swimsuit competition. And I bet you'll have an answer ready when they ask how you'd put an end to world hunger. But you'll still have to balance that heavy crystal crown as you walk down the runway."

She didn't laugh, only smiled politely. She probably doesn't waste her time with silly pop culture, especially something as frivolous as a beauty pageant. Does she even watch TV? I can't imagine there'd be anything on TV that would interest her.

There's something else on her mind. "There are certain countries who do not want me to hold this position, the highest nursing office in the world. Privately, they tell me it's not possible. We won't let you in."

I asked her if it's anti-Semitism, but she waves off that suggestion. "I have no enemies."

I was glad my suspicion was unfounded, but I'm quite sure that if she encountered prejudice of any kind, toward herself or others,

Judith wouldn't hesitate to call it out. "I do not shy from debate," she said. "I'm comfortable with conflict."

"At this stage of my life, my focus is global health, but there are great needs close to home, on our very doorsteps. That's why I'm sending you on this journey. Next week you'll go to Nova Scotia, Newfoundland, New Brunswick, and Ottawa. I'm sending you to VON sites all over Ontario, then out to western Canada to see first-hand the incredible work of the street nurses of Vancouver, where there is the highest incidence of substance abuse in the country. You'll meet a VON nurse who runs a detox unit. You'll spend time with Morag in Edmonton who works in a shelter with women who've experienced domestic violence. Morag is doing research on women who've been strangled during intercourse. You met her at the AGM, right?"

The East Coast! The Rockies! The Prairies! Here I come.

"I want you to visit a First Nations' reserve where the rate of diabetes is five times the national average, where there is the highest rate of cardiac disease, mental illness, suicides, and substance abuse in the entire country. Living conditions are so deplorable there that the people are forced to drink soda pop because it's safer than the water. It is a crisis. You will see all of that when I send you to northern Ontario – Sudbury, North Bay, and Thunder Bay.

Ah, the allure of Thunder Bay. At last, I'll get there.

I leaned back, full of anticipation, excitement, and good food.

I can hardly wait for my adventures to continue, but for now, I return to the present moment. My patient has shown small signs of improvement since the start of my shift this morning. He's more alert, and I've been able to wean down his sedation and a few of the ventilator parameters.

His serious, tight-lipped wife perches at his bedside. There will be many long months of recovery ahead. What will life be like for him at home? She will be his caregiver. What will it be like for her? How will she manage? What supports does she have in place? I try to open a discussion about any concerns she might have, but she shuts it down with a terse, "I'm fine." Perhaps she fears that if she opens up she might break down altogether. I get that. Here, we take care of the most urgent needs. We do today's work today, minute by minute; we don't think about tomorrow. Besides, why would she open up to me? Why invest in a relationship with me? I'm the nurse *du jour*; tomorrow will bring a different one.

My friends want to know when I'll be returning to my regular ICU shifts. "You *are* coming back, aren't you? After you've finished this home care thing? Right?"

Of course I'm coming back, I say, but now, for the first time ever, I'm not so sure.

"There's much to do and we're each responsible for our part," Judith had said after lunch, after I drove her back home and just before she got out of my car.

Her words stayed with me, reverberating like a modern echo of an ancient Talmudic saying: *The day is short and the hours are long. . . . You are not obligated to complete the work, but neither are you free to abandon it.*

Each time I see Judith, I get contemplative about being Jewish. As I drove home after that yummy lunch, I flirted briefly with the possibility of taking my religious observance up a notch. Maybe I'd start going to synagogue more frequently. It couldn't hurt. But definitely not any of the hard-core stuff like refraining from work on the Sabbath or keeping kosher. Yet, what I've always valued even more than the rules carried out to the letter of the law is the moral teachings and the words of wisdom. Judith's beliefs about home care, caregiving, and volunteering reminded me of a passage in the prayer book that I used to hear recited in synagogue when I went with my father.

As soon as I got home, I made a beeline to an old prayer book to look it up. It's called *Eilu D'varim* or "These Are the Things." Reading it again after all these years, I realized that it is not a prayer, but rather a mundane checklist of the basics of human interaction. Honouring elders, welcoming guests, caring for the sick, providing for the needy, celebrating with the bride and groom, comforting the mourner, and being a peacemaker. *These are the things* that connect us to one another, that create community. After all, *life is with people.* And the benefit of following these things (the payback)? *They are beyond all measure.* (Priceless.)

10

FRIED HALIBUT AND RAPPIE PIE

TWENTY-EIGHT YEARS AT VON and you get the feeling she's loved every moment of it.

"I started at the age of ten," Suzanne jokes.

We're sitting in the VON office in Yarmouth, Nova Scotia – the workplace of nurse manager Suzanne D'Entremont, whom I met back in Windsor at the AGM. With her rosy cheeks and a wide, easy smile, she has none of the tense worry lines that I see on the faces of the hospital managers I know. Elegant in a navy suit with a cream-coloured shell and a string of pearls, she's radiant, bubbling over with enthusiasm for her work and for VON.

"This organization helped me grow. When I saw a need for a 'symptom relief kit' to alleviate the discomfort of people dying at home, they gave me the time and resources to develop it. When I had safety concerns about central IV lines, they funded my research. VON has supported my passions – foot health, palliative care, and bereavement support, among others."

Suzanne has organized my itinerary here, a list of clients who receive home care or community supports. She's also arranged for a driver to take me to each place, some of them remote or difficult to find. My driver is Darin Perry, who turns out to be the husband of Janet, the fun-loving executive I met at the AGM who landed in a wheelchair with a sprained ankle after a late night of partying. In fact, Maritimers have a reputation for knowing how to have fun, so it should be an enjoyable trip.

Just as we're about to set out, I ask Suzanne, "I figure about fifteen minutes per visit, right?"

She raises an eyebrow. "I booked you two hours per visit. Stories take time."

We laugh because we both know what it's like in the hospital. There's no time to sit and talk for more than a minute or two with patients. It's more like *shoot, get to the point, cut to the chase, I gotta run.* You'll just get behind in your work and neglect your other patients, or at least they'll feel that way.

"I could never work there. I don't know how you do it," Suzanne says when I tell her where I work. We sit for a few minutes to chat before I set out with Darin to drive to the first visit.

"I worked one year in a hospital," Suzanne says, shaking her head at the memory. "I was so unhappy. Home care is a different culture. It's about relationships and real caring. And as a manager, it has to start with me and trickle down. It's important to me that my staff feel cared about."

They are giving me real caring, too. They've checked me into the local B and B where I'll be staying for the next few days. All I can say about it is that if Prince William and Kate, the Duchess of Cambridge, ever visit Yarmouth, this is where they'd stay. It's as elegant and refined as any royal palace. This morning at breakfast I placed my knife on the silver knife rest – shiny enough to check my lipstick – lifted the lace cover from my linen napkin, and was confronted with the perplexing choice of a warm pumpkiň spice muffin or a banana muffin with my morning coffee. The owner, Twyla, has already run ten kilometres, showered and dressed, then bathed and dressed her special needs foster child, Wendy, and tended to a sick dog. She's also folded laundry, ironed bed sheets (!), and made a delicious breakfast, including per-fectly poached eggs and toast from homemade bread, plus the aforementioned muffins. When I compliment her baking she runs to print a copy of the recipe for the muffin I chose.

After breakfast, Darin and I get into the car and he takes us along a quiet scenic highway, then some twisty country roads. We've left the rich, fertile Annapolis Valley and are now near the most western tip of Nova Scotia. He turns onto a dirt road, at the end of which is a little lake and the cutest little blue-trimmed clapboard house with two pumpkins on the front steps. It belongs to Sandra, her husband, Leon, and Sandra's daughter Cheryl, who has a rare genetic disorder called Alström Syndrome.

"There are only eight hundred cases in the world. Same as the number of pandas," Cheryl tells me proudly. Sandra has become an authority on this condition and she describes the effects on the eyes, ears, heart, and kidneys that Cheryl, now eighteen, has developed: obesity, diabetes, scoliosis, and now, cardiac problems, which Cheryl is beginning to develop.

Cheryl sits in a wing chair beside Leon. She wears a Pink "Le Shopping" sweatshirt, grey baggy sweatpants, and sunglasses because of photophobia and limited vision. "I see lights and darks – just like laundry," she jokes. Recently, she was diagnosed with a serious heart problem that is well controlled on cardiac medications, but may worsen in time.

"There's nothing to do all day," Cheryl grumbles, "so I have to stay home with him." She points a thumb at Leon, her stepfather, who looks amused at her comment and smiles lovingly at her. "I spend all day in my 'upstairs zone,' my loft."

Sandra picked up the early signs of Cheryl's condition.

"At nine months, her eyes started wobbling. The ophthalmologist said it was nothing, but my gut told me otherwise. Behind his back, the medical intern called to say, 'I could get in trouble, but I disagree with him.' He suggested we get a second opinion and an ERG, an electro-retinogram. Sure enough, Cheryl has no cones or rods."

Cheryl picks up there. "School was okay, but some kids were mean and made fun of me. When I was thirteen, I went to Halifax to a school for the blind, but I prefer to be alone. I don't fit in the outside world. I'm a puzzle piece that can't find its place."

She gets up, slowly, and makes her way up to her room to get something to show me. In her brief absence, Sandra can say things that are hard to say in front of Cheryl, even though there are no secrets here. They have given me permission to write about everything, and of course Cheryl will read it, too. "We don't hide anything," Sandra says. "Cheryl's personality is difficult and she knows it. She's stubborn, always has to have the last word. Motherhood was different than what I expected. There's a poem I read once about going to Holland. You're expecting wooden shoes, windmills, and tulips, but you land up in Italy with fountains and cathedrals. It turns out to be a positive experience, but it wasn't at all what you expected. I was devastated. Even now, every year at prom time, I get choked up, knowing what Cheryl and I are missing out on. We're definitely attached at the hip. She and Leon tease each other, but she adores him and he's crazy about her. It's been a challenge to be her mother and her caregiver. Emotionally she's a teenager, but at times, she likes to be in her childhood years with her Wiggles and Muppets and Teletubbies. On the other hand, she is mature, wise beyond her years. She doesn't like going to her father but she understands Leon and I need our time together. She'll say, 'You two go have a shower together. Get the romance thing going again.' She gets it."

Cheryl returns and plunks herself down into her chair. She opens a copy of *Anne of Green Gables*, turns to a random page, and slowly moves her fingertips horizontally across the long white pages of raised dots ("I'm not a speed reader, you know," she warns me in case I happen to be impatient) and reads aloud. "'What a splendid day!' said Anne, drawing a long breath. 'Isn't it good just to be alive on a day like this? I pity the people who aren't born yet for missing it.'" Cheryl slams the book shut. "With my condition, I need a lot of sleep. After breakfast, I go back to bed or spend the day on the computer. I'm very isolated. I hate my life. I have no friends. I'm stuck here with Leon all day." Cheryl scowls in his direction and Leon smiles back at her from where he sits in an easy chair, working on a crossword puzzle.

"What do you like to do? Any hobbies?" I ask.

"I have nothing to do but sit here by myself."

"What about singing?" Sandra reminds her. "Cheryl likes to sing," she tells me.

"Yes, but I won't go in the choir."

"Cheryl has a hearing impairment. She wears a hearing aid."

"Yeah and when you call out, 'Your sandwich is ready!' it's so loud." Cheryl covers her ears.

"Cheryl's in good health," Sandra says, "but needs close monitoring to keep her well."

"I have a hard life." Cheryl casts her eyes down to her lap.

"Cheryl's been a blessing," Sandra says to me, then looks at her. "You've taught me so much."

"Like what?" Cheryl looks up at her mother.

"How to see not just with the eyes."

"How can I teach *you* to see when I can't see?"

"You've taught me how to see with my heart. You've taught me courage and resilience."

"Because of my low vision, I have to rely on my imagination," Cheryl explains to me.

I tell her she reminds me of the Bubble Boy on a *Seinfeld* episode. Like her, he was isolated, had a rare disease, devoted parents – cranky and smart, too, with a sharp wit and caustic tongue.

"I don't watch *Seinfeld*. I like the *Big Bang Theory*."

Cheryl gets up to retreat to her loft, allowing Sandra to speak even more openly.

"What's the hardest part?" I ask her.

"For me, it's self-care. When I'm at my worst, trying to juggle work, Cheryl's care, and thinking about the impending loss of her – because we know her condition will get worse – I feel guilty doing things that are just for me, like exercising, meditation, sitting with friends. And eating properly is so difficult. She's my daughter and I love her, so why do I lose patience? At times I feel I don't have a life to myself. I'm a sentry, always on duty."

"How do you deal with the thought of losing her?"

"The cardiac problems are a new worry. 'This might take you early,' I told her in a very concrete way. She says she wants to be buried in a pink dress, with her four Wiggle dolls. I didn't think she really got it until one day, out of the blue, she said, 'I'm worried I'm going to die.' I told her, 'I'm worried, too, but I'll be there with you.' It was a freeing moment for both of us because it wasn't a secret anymore. What a relief."

Sandra loves talking about her daughter. "Cheryl's smart. She has an extraordinary memory for numbers, dates, events. She does accents, Australian, Italian, Scottish – she does an amazing Shrek and Donkey. Can recite long stretches of dialogue. It's like pushing a Play button on a tape recorder and it all comes out."

A few years ago, Sandra studied to become a therapist and sees private clients and couples in her office. She shows me her business card with her motto printed on it: "Let's talk about it." How apt. She's so easy to talk to it's difficult to say goodbye, but we have to move on.

From the car, I gaze out at the beautiful, soothing coastline while Darin does the driving.

Next, I meet Don and Betty Smith in their tiny bungalow in which every inch of space is an expression of their life together on the sea – a clock in the shape of a lighthouse, shell-studded picture frames, light switches with sails, a mirror set in a barometer case, a thermometer wrapped in nautical knots. Together, they fished for almost thirty years, until Don's stroke a year ago changed all of that.

Betty is in her eighties and Don's almost ninety. Even though he's sitting in a deep chair, I can see he's a tall man. And I notice how scrubbed clean and meticulously dressed he is, in pressed flannel pyjamas, a soft red-plaid lumber jacket, leather moccasins with fur lining. As for Betty, I'd be surprised if she weighs eighty pounds, but whatever the scales say, it's all muscle. Don's way over six feet, she tells me, and she's almost five feet – yet you get the feeling she could lift a truck, a dory, even haul a whale out of the water if she had to, that there's nothing she couldn't do or wouldn't at least try. She tells me that she operated the fishing boat by herself and that in her kayak she paddled far out into the ocean, as recently as a year ago. Now, caring for Don is a full-time job, but she loves to tell stories about the good old days and he enjoys listening.

"What did you do for fun?"

"Oh, lots of things. We made our own bread. We went mossing."

She explains that Irish moss is an edible herb, like the fiddleheads, nettles, and sorrel they also foraged for. "We made perfume and ice cream from it. We'd stand up in the dory and haul the stuff onto the boat with long rakes. Hard work, but we were content. That way of life is over now," Betty says, her smile wistful. "We made do with little. My kids never had toys or birthday parties, but they were happy. Fishing was how we made our living. It was the only life we knew. Whatever the weather, we went out to sea, but the younger generation isn't interested in that life."

Don hasn't moved or spoken but seems to be listening to our conversation.

"How do you manage with caring for Don?"

Betty springs into action to demonstrate how she pumps the hydraulic mechanism of the mechanical lifter to transfer Don from the bed to the chair and back to bed in the evening, but quickly returns to her favourite topic – his, too, by the smile on his face.

"Oh, those were wonderful days! Our children swam in the icy ocean water, played together, everyone. I fished beside Don for twenty-five years and raised five kids on the island."

"She grew up the kids on her own," Don says in a slow voice, his speech slurred.

"I was the hired man, sat in the stern. Don was the captain, and the fisherman, always. We halibutted, swordfished, lobstered, dragged for flounder. In Clark's Harbour and on Cape Sable Island, in summer, fall, and spring. Everything was done by hand. Halibut are huge fish. I don't know how I had the strength to pull them in. Our hands were cut up and rough. At night, I'd wash Don's hands in hot, soapy water, then soak them in baby oil."

I kneel beside Don and pick up his massive, heavy hands and turn them over to examine them. There are more stories here than a fortune teller could read, but it's now up to Betty to tell the tales of his hands and their life together on the sea.

"Nowadays, they have heaters on their boats. We didn't have that back then, oh no. Old boats didn't have a shelter; you were exposed. One time a helicopter had to drop us food and coal."

"How did you keep warm?"

"Hard work. Kept on moving. Never stopped. That's how you keep the blood flowing. For me, an hour working outdoors is better than any medication."

"What bait do lobsters like?" I turn to Don.

"Herr . . . ing, mack . . . erel," he starts slowly, and it's Betty to the rescue.

"We also trawled and hand-lined for cod. Those were fun times, even with all the accidents – one with an outboard motor. His hand was bleeding like stink. Two weeks later we went back to shore – it was fourteen miles from land – had it x-rayed and found two fractures."

"Betty jerry-rigged . . . something to make a . . . splint for me," Don manages to get out.

"We set up a fishing camp, started out early each morning, depending on the tides and winds. Had five children, home-schooled them on the island, but they had to have French, so for that they had to go to school on the mainland. Now, I have twelve grandchildren and twelve great-grandchildren. Then, one day, I was sawing wood with the weed-whacker when Don said, 'Something's wrong. I can't move.' So we brought him to land and indeed it was a stroke. Then, a few days later, he had another stroke in the brain stem. When they brought him home from the hospital, they put him in the bed, propped him up with pillows and said, 'He's all yours.' It was up to me. He couldn't walk, but in six weeks, he was up on his feet. The kids and I, we make him reach for things. I tied a rope around his foot so he can pull his leg up. Every morning we get up at half past four and right away I start exercising him so he don't get stiff. Everything we do is part of his therapy. Everyone stays positive. Even the cable guy who came to fix the TV was encouraging. I never say you can't do anything. I always say you can. You have to try."

Every morning Betty bathes Don, dresses him, takes him to the bathroom, and gets him into his wheelchair for breakfast. In her spare time, she makes quilts. She jumps up to run to her sewing room and returns in an instant with an armful of handmade, cheerful quilts with blocks of maple leaf, cathedral windows, churn dash, and pineapples, all made from old clothes. She shows me her garden where she grows potatoes, peas, lettuce, and flowers — gladiolas and dahlias.

Her daughter Leona drops for a visit. Betty whispers to me, "Leona's a dear, but a worrier."

Leona sits down in the closest seat, her Dad's wheelchair. "I just live down the street and am always popping in to check on them, to make sure they're okay. I worry about them all the time." She joins her mom and dad in their reminiscences of life on the sea. "I liked being a Capie. I've grown up all my life along the water. I know the dangers. My brother has been overboard twice. Every male in this family is on the water at the start of lobster season. I knew people who've drowned. We know if a boat is missing. You're always listening to the CB radio to hear if the boat's been found."

Leona looks anxious but Betty is fearless. At eighty-five she still drives and stays active in the community. "I take Don to the day program, then I run a few errands and go to the caregiver support group. Some people there had to put their spouse in a nursing home and feel bad about it. But they had no choice. They had Alzheimer's and were wandering or aggressive. Don wouldn't get far, and if he tried to beat up on me, I'd give it right back." He looks at her fondly and tries to smile, but is unable to fully activate the muscles in his partially paralyzed face.

"How long do you think you'll be able to take care of Don by yourself?" I ask Betty.

"It depends on my health. Once, I fell on top of him and broke my wrist, but I managed to pick him up. He's forgetful but I am, too. I guess at our age it's allowed. The day program is so good for him and for me, too. At first, he didn't want to go, but now he likes going."

"What's your favourite thing to do there?" I ask Don.

"Play . . . poker with the girls. I don't want . . . to go to one of those death places," he manages to say, attempting to grin.

"That's how he calls the nursing home," Betty says. "I hope to keep him home."

"When I wake . . . up in the morning, I wiggle my fingers and squeeze my hand to get . . . the circulation going. I dream I'm still . . . out on the boat with the guys, then I realize . . . they're dead and I'm still alive. What are . . . you going to do? Life . . . goes on until it stops, don't it?"

There's no other place for Betty to be but beside him, and for him but beside her.

It's time to move on. Reluctantly, I get up and say goodbye. I take another glance around as I leave. No one does homespun coziness like Maritimers. They decorate with a sense of home as a refuge, a place for comfort as well as shelter, a haven you'd never want to leave. Perhaps it comes from an awareness that life is tough, so at least at home you are comfortable and safe.

The VON office is the hub of all of our visits, so Darin drives us back there to get the next address and set of directions from Suzanne. It's like we're on the *Amazing Race* – Team Darin dashes in to a pit stop, gets new instructions, and we race to the next destination. But once we arrive at each visit, I slow down, quiet my mind, and remind myself of what Suzanne said: *stories take time.*

As we drive to the next visit, we pass farmhouses, where all the porches have easy chairs, set up in position for conversations, as if inviting you to stop and sit awhile. We drive on Ye Olde Argyle Road, a twisting country lane along the coast. The ocean is a constant backdrop and the landscape is dotted with green, blue, and white farmhouses nestled in among the trees in their glorious fall colours. As we drive past the edge of the Bay of Fundy, Darin points out where the tides come in by late afternoon. "Whoosh!" he says with a sweep of his arm. "A tidal bore comes in one big wave, all at once. If you're not careful, you'll be stranded. These tides can beat a racehorse."

At the next house, I can't tell who's more bursting with pride, the client or his nurse.

Ken looks like a shrunken Hulk Hogan, the same rugged, manly face, a wide, solid frame, big blue eyes, and nicely trimmed blond beard. He waves his cane over at Nurse Charline. "It's because of her." Charline sits back in an easy chair, beaming at what they accomplished together.

Four years ago, Ken was mowing the grass barefoot, clearing out the bramble, and got scratches from blackberry bushes. His heels got infected and wouldn't heal. The infection spread all along his legs. "It quickly got to the point where I couldn't walk. Couldn't wear shoes."

Three times a day for two years, then two times a day for two years, Charline applied dressings, ointments, compression bandages, and helped him get his diet, weight, blood pressure, and blood sugar levels under control. Diabetics heal slowly, sometimes not at all, so it took that much time, plus their perseverance and partnership.

"Yup, she fixed me up real good. She prayed for me and lit candles at church."

"Surely she did more than that," I tease him.

"She's a kind person, for sure. Smart, too." He grins at his partner.

"I had a dream about your legs last night, Ken," Charline says affectionately.

"Ain't that something . . ."

"See, I'd been a bouncer at the casino on the reserve, but it got so I couldn't walk. I had to quit my job. I had no choice but to go to a doctor. For me, that's like having a tooth extracted without anesthesia. That doctor sent me to a whatchamacallit . . ."

"A vascular surgeon," Charline says.

"He told me point-blank, 'These wounds will not heal. The only solution is amputation.' *Let me outta here,* I thought. I don't want to live my life in a wheelchair. It struck a nerve. I started doing what Charline told me."

"You see, Ken hadn't been taking good care of himself," Charline explains. "For starters, he was overweight. Now, that's a problem I have, too, but it helped me understand him better than a thin nurse might." Ken also smoked and had poor circulation, sleep apnea, and arterial and venous leg blockages that prevented his legs from healing. "They drained constantly, some days more than a litre. I soaked them twice daily in saline and we tried various ointments – antibacterial, zinc, even honey. His legs were super-sensitive. Elevating his legs helped, but it was too painful. We helped him learn to balance his sugar and got him onto a better diet."

"Tell her about the surprise you found. The creepy crawlers." Ken cues her.

"It was a hot summer day. I'd been here in the morning and his legs were fine, but at the afternoon visit, I couldn't believe my eyes – they were covered in maggots. It turned out to be a good thing because they ate the dead tissue, left the healing skin alone, and did their work painlessly."

"Miracle maggots, they were."

"His legs look great now," Charline says. "Show her our masterpiece," she prompts him.

Ken takes off his shoes and socks and stands up for my close inspection. His legs are thin, scarred and discoloured, but I see no signs of infection. The pulses are strong and easy to palpate. Best of all, he can slip on his new shoes and walk.

"Without Charline, I wouldn't have a leg to stand on – literally. Now, I drive, work part-time as prep cook at the diner down the road. It's all because of her." He points with his cane at his nurse. "Charline saved my legs."

"Seeing Ken's legs heal, now wearing his shoes, it's like watching my own baby take his first steps. It's been the most rewarding experience of my career. There's a chance of recurrence so I drop by once a week to check on him, but soon he won't need me anymore."

"It will be hard for me when Charline gives me the heave-ho."

I have a feeling it will be hard for her, too. Their love is mutual, yet entirely professional. It's part admiration, part awe. I've never seen a patient and nurse as closely bonded, as united as Ken and Charline have been on their mission to save Ken's legs.

Darin drops me off in a clinic parking lot and zooms off. He'll pick me up later after my visits with Nurse Claudette. She's waiting for me at the front entrance to a little clinic that sits right on the ocean shore. "This is my supply cupboard," she says and pops open the trunk of her car. It's jam-packed with boxes of catheters, gauze, vinyl gloves, and more. She tells me about her client we're about to see. Mink is morbidly obese – over six hundred pounds, by my estimation – and needs wound care that he couldn't possibly manage by himself, given his bulk.

"Why do you meet him at this clinic, not at his home?" I ask Claudette.

"We used to go to his home, but Mink runs a bootleg operation, making moonshine. 'The Establishment,' he calls it. There were *transactions* going on when the nurses would visit, so we told him he had to come here for his dressing changes. He complains about it, but don't you worry about Mink," Claudette says. "He's got a nice life and is richer than you or me. Has an attractive lady friend, to boot. Bee takes care of him, drives him around, gets him groceries."

"What are you going to do for him today?"

"I'm going to change the dressings on his wounds on his legs, groin, and buttocks. You see, Mink can't reach his feet or his back. He has a urinary catheter and a huge penis."

A huge penis? Why is that relevant?

"Why does Mink have a catheter?" I ask, my mind considering the usual possibilities, like renal failure or urethral obstruction. It turns out to be not as complicated as that. It's pure body mechanics, as Claudette explains.

"He can't reach his penis over his belly, and it's hidden deep inside the folds of fat and won't come out. Urine gets in there and he can't keep it clean. There is also a hygiene issue."

While Bee waits for him out in the reception area, we go in to meet Mink.

"They removed a ninety-pound tumour," Mink tells me right off the bat.

"Mink is referring to his weight-loss surgery," Claudette clarifies. "You underwent a *pannectomy*," she reminds him.

Then it dawns on me: Claudette's Quebecois accent made "pannus" – the medical term for the apron of fat around Mink's gut – sound like "penis." That's what she was describing as so "huge." Indeed, Mink's belly droops down to his knees. Giant pantaloons of adipose tissue hang at the back of his legs. "The surgeons tried to remove them but there was *hemorrhage*," Claudette explains, her beautiful accent making that word sound like the name of a French perfume. She helps Mink haul himself up onto the treatment table where he spreads his legs to expose extensive surgical and pressure wounds in his abdomen, groin, and inner thighs. Claudette examines them closely and draws comparisons to the last time she saw them, observing the depth, shape, and drainage from each one. She takes off the soiled dressings, cleans the wounds, and begins a long process of applying new dressings and attaching some of them to a suction machine to improve drainage.

"Every two weeks we change his catheter. Today, it just needs to be irrigated."

I help her lift the folds of fat so that she can insert the catheter. *How would she ever do this procedure all by herself?* "First I have to find it," she says.

Mink grins and chuckles. "Did the hedgehog go into the cave?"

"In the ICU we call that *turtle-itis*," I tell him.

After the dressing change, Claudette and I give Mink a bath, scrubbing him with buckets of soapy water and using long, broad strokes, like we're washing a car. Claudette dries off one side of him with a large bath towel and I dry off the other. We help him get dressed, then ease him down off the stretcher and onto his feet. He seems to feel pampered by that routine, but tiny beads of perspiration have collected on Claudette's forehead and upper lip. It was hard physical labour. *How does she manage to do this all on her own?*

Mink loops the electrical cord from the wound suction machine around his neck. It will run on battery until he gets home and can plug it in. Already, cloudy drainage is trickling into the new collection chamber that Claudette's just installed.

"How's the diet coming along?" Claudette asks as she washes her hands and arms up to her elbows, at the sink.

"Good, good," he says with an evasive wave. He hikes up his track pants and ties the rubber skipping rope that he uses as a belt.

"Tell us what you've been eating."

"Well . . . I'm not a salad man." He gives a sly grin. "I eat yogurt and grapes. Mostly."

Claudette helps him up onto the veterinary scale once used for farm livestock. They keep it in the clinic just for Mink. She balances the weights.

"Well, you must be doing something right. You lost two pounds."

"Do you cook for yourself, Mink? Does Bee?" I ask.

"No, she can't cook, but I make a mean rabbit stew."

"Just out of curiosity, what goes in a rabbit stew?" *Elmer Fudd wants to make a wabbit stew.*

"Carrots, of course."

"Yes. That makes sense."

"Soya sauce, too. It kills the taste of wild. Onion, too, sometimes."

We go out to the waiting room to join Bee and discuss the recipe further.

"Pshaw!" Bee exclaims. "Don't listen to him, the old coot. Onion in rabbit stew? Never! Say, if you come to visit us, we'll make you pease pudding and blueberry duff."

"Yeah, and stuffed cat, a roast chicken with dressing and a bit of arsenic thrown in."

"How do you manage with chores like cooking and cleaning?" I ask.

"I toss leftovers and garbage up onto the roof for the seagulls."

Afterwards, back at the car, I have to ask Claudette the question any hospital nurse would ask.

"Mink seems so dependent on the nurses. Couldn't he do more for himself?"

"We are working with him to get him to take more ownership of his care, but he's resistant."

"That wouldn't go over well in the hospital. We push people to do as much self-care as they possibly can, perhaps before they're ready, but in the belief that it's best for them. How does it help him to do everything for him?"

"We've made small steps of progress. He now brings clean clothes to change into or we won't wash him. It's a start. We accept him as he is." She sees I'm not convinced. Not many hospital nurses would be. But then, Claudette shares something about Mink that we probably wouldn't have an opportunity to know in the hospital.

"Mink's had a rough life. His father sexually abused him. His step-father physically abused him. He'd leave him outside in the winter, and duct-taped him to a chair when he was inside. The kindness he receives from the nurses is new for him. It's the only kindness he's ever known."

Once you know a person's story, you're not as quick to judge.

Claudette drives us to her next client – Pierre, a sixty-five-year-old widower with bowel cancer and a recent colostomy. When Claudette removes the bag, it's like the smell of shame fills the bathroom, and he gets tearful. They speak quietly in French, but I get the gist.

"I want to stay home," Pierre says. "I don't want to go to . . . a . . . one of those *places.*"

"As long as you have a bit of help, you can manage at home?"

"I know it smells like shit, but it's my shit and it's my home." Claudette nods and they share a quiet laugh. Magically, she's managed to normalize the bizarre situation of having liquid stool trickle – sometimes gush – out of a hole in one's abdomen and into a bag glued to one's body. As she cleans the skin and places the new bag, she asks about his mood, energy, and appetite. *She treats Pierre as a whole, not just his hole.* I can see how this kind of nursing helps people cope with life, not just with illness.

In the evening, Darin and Suzanne take me out for a delicious meal of halibut, shrimp, scallops, and lobster, straight from the sea. Even when I'm full, and couldn't possibly eat another thing, they insist I try the local specialty, *râpure*, an Acadian dish made of potatoes, cheese, and sometimes chicken, too. Well, I'm always up for a challenge, especially one involving food.

Mmm . . . I could get hooked on this smooth, creamy comfort food.

They joke that there are only a few surnames in Yarmouth, because everyone is related to one another. D'Eon, Saulnier, Daignealt, Boudreau, Joudrey, and D'Entremont are exotic to me, but common here. It's a small town, so even those not related by blood seem like relatives due to the close involvement in each other's lives.

As we get up to go, I'm glad I don't have to say goodbye just yet. Suzanne has planned a special event for tomorrow evening, so I'll see her then.

Darin drives me to the B and B. I sit in the back seat, deep in thought, thinking about feet. It's a subject that has, well, legs. "I'm determined that people go to their graves with both limbs," Suzanne had said fervently, like it was a prayer.

"Instead of amputations and rehabilitation, let's keep people on their feet. Most people don't think much about the health of their feet. Perhaps they feel it's beneath them." We laughed at her unintended pun. "In our society, we have an aversion to feet, but I always think about Jesus washing the feet of the poor and the humility that implies. That image inspires me."

It's true. We pay so much attention to hearts, livers, and lungs. Rightly so. You can't live without those organs, yet what's a life if you lose your feet? Sure, if you're born without feet or lose them when you're still young and healthy, you can get a prosthesis and adapt, but what if you're older and dealing with impaired health already? I've often heard it said that prevention isn't exciting because, when done right, nothing happens; yet that's exactly what should happen to healthy feet. Nothing. In fact, when Darin asks what I'm so deep in thought about, I'm too tired to explain, so that's exactly what I answer.

"Nothing."

Guest-Lovitt House B & B
   Yarmouth, Nova Scotia

Twyla's Banana Muffins

3 large or 4 small ripe bananas mashed in a small bowl
In another bowl, mix:
3/4 cup white sugar
1 1/2 cups flour (half whole wheat and half white)
1 tsp baking powder
1 tsp baking soda
1/2 tsp salt
1 egg
1/3 cup oil
1 tsp vanilla
Add banana, 1/4 cup walnuts, and 1/2 cup chocolate chips
Bake at 375 degrees for 20 minutes

   Hope you enjoy!

11

YOU SAY GOODBYE, I SAY HELLO

"FROM HERE, YOU CAN SEE THE BRIDGE that takes you all the way over to Prince Edward Island." Darin points to the far shore. I can barely make that out in the dense early morning fog, much less the bridge to P.E.I.

"So you're not just my driver. You're my tour guide, too," I say, but he pays no notice to my teasing. He's focused on the land and the sea he loves.

"If you squint — or have a wicked good imagination — you can almost see the red earth potato fields."

"What about the red braids belonging to Anne of Green Gables? Can you see those, too? What about her house in Avonlea?"

"Aww . . . you tourists are all the same. Once, I took a visitor over there who had to see Anne's house. Then she asked to go to the cemetery to visit her grave! I had to break her heart and tell her the truth. But P.E.I. is beautiful. It's so tiny, you can walk across the entire province in an hour, drive across in two minutes." He tells me they turn the porch lights on and off at night to confuse ships, but I think he's kidding about that.

———

Our first stop is at Henrietta Denby's tidy little pink house with a flower garden overlooking the sea. We sit in her front "parlour," where I drink tea and listen.

"I never felt ready or prepared, but I've been called upon to be a caregiver my whole life. My caregiving career started at sixteen when my grandmother lived with us – my parents, brothers, and sisters. She had Alzheimer's and I shared my bedroom with her. My mother was busy with the other kids, so I did all of the hands-on care for her. She would dirty herself and hide the you-know-what. We had no outside help. We did it all ourselves." We both take a sip of our tea. She settles in her chair, takes a few moments, and then gets to the story she really wants to tell.

"My husband, Coleman, died last year. Two years prior, he had been diagnosed at sixty-four with multiple myeloma – and yes, we dreamed of getting older, getting to sixty-four together, just like in the Beatles song." As Henrietta speaks, her pensive face and frequent pauses make me feel she is reliving it. The pain of remembering crosses her face, but then she collects herself and continues. "I was just thinking about his pain. Deep, searing bone pain. Horrific pain. They wanted to send us straight to palliative care but Coleman opted for aggressive treatment. Let me tell you, chemo is no walk in the park. He had every complication – nausea, mouth sores, infections, pneumonia.

"One morning he awoke screaming. It was his neck. The tumour had pushed through his vertebrae. He was in terrible pain. Luckily, I remembered we had a cervical collar in the closet and I ran to get it. The ambulance came and took him to the hospital. The doctors told us all along that the treatment was not to cure it, but to stave it off for as long as possible. Then they offered us to be in a clinical trial for thalidomide. That scared us. We only knew of that drug from bad stories growing up, but it helped – for awhile. He accepted his fate, but it took me a lot longer to do so. When he realized he wasn't going to get better, he was the one to tell me. He began to prepare me for his death."

"How did he do that?"

"He was a carpenter and appreciated the craftsmanship of old buildings. He'd saved doors and window frames. He organized his door collection for our son. He prepared a detailed blueprint of the house so I could maintain it. He was a big-boys-don't-cry type but his actions said it all. Not big on words, but I always felt loved. We had a nest egg, but we had to dip into it and that worried him. One of the drugs he was on was experimental and it wasn't covered. It was expensive and he didn't want to deplete our savings and what would be left for me.

"We went through it all together. We're not overly religious, but we did daily readings and prayers that gave us comfort. One was about a mother eagle, pushing her baby from the nest. It was exactly how I felt. From then on, we kept spotting eagles. Each time I thought, There goes my eagle. I'll be okay. I see so many eagles now. Were they always there but only now I see them? Perhaps. Coleman was the fixer in our life, the protector, for me, our children, but we couldn't fix him.

"Toward the end was when the real conversations began. He said to me one day, 'Henny, you have to realize that I'm not going to get well.' I was still in denial. He helped me face the reality. Until then, denial had been useful, but it was time to let it go. We planned for him to go into hospice. He thought it would be unpleasant for the grandchildren and too much work for me if he died at home. He was always protecting us, especially me, and he was proud and didn't want the children to see him like that.

"Then came a day when we had no choice; he had to go into the hospital. The pain was unbearable. They got his pain under control, but the meds made him drowsy all the time and also more confused and not with us as much. Easter was coming and I asked him if he wanted to come home that day, just for the day. So he celebrated Easter and then we made the decision that he wouldn't go back to the hospital. 'Can you do this?' he asked me. He wanted to be home, but only if I could handle it. 'I can die at home if you are able to care for me.' I didn't know and I was scared, but the home care nurses came in and taught me. They empowered me. Without them there was no way we could have done it. They taught my children to give the meds. They were with us every step of the way. I was a layperson – what did I know about Hickman lines and portacaths? One night the battery ran out on his medication pump. I was afraid it would block off and we wouldn't be able to give him pain medication. I called the nurse and in the middle of the night she came over. It was so overwhelming, all of it. It was hard having so many people at the house. He was a private person and very proud. He didn't want anyone to see him like that. I pleaded with God. Heal him or take him.

"It was November 11, Remembrance Day. Coleman was an old soldier, a veteran of the Cuban missile crisis, and he wanted to watch the memorial service on the TV in the living room. We managed to get him there, but suddenly he said, 'I want to go back to bed.' He was one hundred pounds but a dead weight. Just as my son and I were carrying him across the living room, to the bedroom, he stopped us. 'Wait,' he said. 'Let me look around. I won't see this living room again.' He was right. He knew. We were all with him at the end. Rose, our daughter, read him a poem she wrote and many people came to say goodbye. The grandchildren brought written messages for him that we read aloud. Some of the children were frightened and wanted to run away, but the nurses made them feel comfortable and helped them stay, even gave them little tasks to do, like massaging his feet or suctioning the secretions in his mouth. I sat by his bed and read him the love poems that I had written to him over the past weeks. I was able to thank him for all that he was and all that he had given us. I went from loving him to cherishing him. Everyone came and said their goodbyes.

"It was November 13. He didn't speak all day. By then, he was getting morphine 'round the clock. There were times when he was short of breath, but the nurses told us not to panic and just calmly give the morphine if they weren't there to do it. Mostly, we knew exactly how much to give and when, but I was scared I might give the fatal dose. But when I saw it from his point of view, I realized the morphine was a kindness. It wasn't about me, it was about what *he* needed."

She pauses for a few minutes and dries her eyes with a pressed handkerchief. We sip our tea and soon she is ready – and eager – to tell me more.

"It's so hard to stand by and not do anything, to make that switch from cure to care. Mostly, he was comfortable and alert. When I gave him a bath near the end, I knew it was his last. I used nice soap and warm water – none of that chemical stuff they put on him in the hospital. That bath helped me let him go. A feeling of peace washed over me. Later that day his doctor, Dr. Leahey, came and asked him, "'Coleman, how are you feeling?' He said, 'I'm on top of the world.' 'What do you mean?' He said, 'You know.' At the end, she said to me, 'A job well done.' It meant so much to me, coming from her, a doctor Coleman respected so much."

"How are you doing now?" I mean both right now in this moment, having relived that painful time, and also now, in this new chapter in her life. I leave it to her to take either meaning.

"I yearn to feel his body, to hear his voice. At times I'm angry. Mostly I feel forsaken. I felt lonesome, but not for anyone. For Coleman. Friends don't know what to say. They don't call or come over because they're afraid of disturbing me – or perhaps themselves. When he slept so much in the last few months, I had thoughts of all of our plans and dreams, but I knew none of that would happen."

She shows me a picture of them, taken a few weeks before he died.

"He was handsome," I say. As for Henrietta, she appeared tense and haggard. Coleman was smiling broadly; she, not at all. She's looking much better now, but clearly his dying was harder on her than on him.

"His dying was agonizing for me, but I made sure it wasn't for him. But if the nurses hadn't prepared me, it would have been traumatic. They told me exactly what to expect, what dying actually entails, the gurgling sounds, the smells, the erratic breathing, gasping at the end."

"It's distressing if you've never seen it before."

"It's not easy to turn your house into a hospital, but for the comfort of having him at home and being with him all the time it was worth it."

"I've cared for many dying people, but I've rarely seen a natural, peaceful death like that. You should feel very proud that you were able to give that gift to Coleman."

"Afterwards, I was never more exhausted. I felt like I'd run a marathon."

"You had. You deserve an honorary degree."

"In what?"

"In caregiving."

"We couldn't have done it without the nurses. They weren't just nurses, they were teachers. They showed us how to do everything, explained what was happening, what would happen. I've since learned that most people don't have that kind of beautiful death."

We sit quietly for a few minutes, until Henrietta is ready to speak. "I love fall. I feel him around me at this time of year. You know, I still see eagles from time to time."

"I hope his last few months of dying isn't all bad memories for you," I say.

"Not at all." She smiles. "We had laughs, even during that time. One day, I was bent down, tying his shoes. 'I bet you never thought you'd be tying my shoes,' he said. 'It's a lot better than wiping your butt,' I said. But then the day came that I had to wipe his butt, and as I was doing that, he said, 'I bet you wish you were tying my shoes.' Well, we both totally lost it. We never laughed so hard." Henrietta pauses to smile at that happy memory.

Henrietta has started volunteering at the hospital. She's beginning to get into her new life.

There's something else she wants to tell me.

"A few weeks after he died, I came across a note tucked into a little dollar store tray I keep on my dresser. He'd wanted me to find it after he was gone. 'One of the greatest blessings God can give is a spouse that loves you and you love in return.' That said it all. It was so typical of our marriage." She dabs at her eyes and apologizes. "Then, just a few months ago, my wedding ring was tight and I'd been meaning to remove it. On our anniversary date, suddenly, the ring loosened on its own and I didn't have to cut it off. See, he's still looking after me."

Now the tears flow and she lets them, and I can't help myself – I join her. "What can I do? I've lost my true love. We found each other in high school and we never let go. He taught me how to love. Yes, I will live on and I will love until I can love no longer."

On the road to our next stop, I scan the sky for eagles before dropping off for a power nap, another of my sleeping talents. After a few minutes, I wake up refreshed and look out the window. Farmland on the left, the sea on the right.

"Oh, look," I say, "horses."

"Here in the Maritimes, we call them cows."

I put on my glasses for a closer look. Peering out my window, I see that they are indeed bovines, grazing peacefully in a meadow. "Oh. I see what you mean."

He smiles at me in his rear-view mirror. "You really are a city slicker." He points out some black and white cows in a field. "Those are Oreo cows. You'll only find those in the Maritimes. See how the neck and rump are dark chocolate and the middle third is vanilla?"

"In the hospital, we have cows, too," I tease him back. "Computers on Wheels."

Soon, we arrive at the nursing home where the chief administrator – a chic, petite blond woman, looking glamorous in a beige Chanel-type suit and high heels – meets me at the front door with a smile and a disconcerting greeting: "Hi, I'm Bertha, the Death Woman." She leads me to her office. It's an oasis of calm with stained glass windows on the door, polished wood floors, and the peaceful stillness of a chapel – which is, in fact, what it was before Bertha Brannen made it into her workspace.

Bertha's specialty is death, dying, and mourning. She organizes bereavement support groups, which grew in logical sequence from the caregiver support groups that VON had already established in the area. Bertha conducts divorce groups, too, because she believes there are a lot of similarities between grieving the loss of a loved one and grieving the loss of a marriage. I ask her about how she became interested in topics most people would rather not think about.

"My sister died at the age of twenty-five. Alice was so *baaaad*. We all had blond hair and she alone had dark. 'I'm Elvis's love child,' she'd say. Oh, she had a devilish sense of humour. My mother died a few years later, at the age of forty-seven. When you're facing death, your own or someone you love, you are honest.

"We are a death-denying society. In the past, widows wore black. A wreath was hung on the front door. The coffin stayed in the house. The community gathered to offer support. Now, we rush it along. Drive-through grief. I asked a friend how someone whose husband had recently died was doing. 'Not well. She's sad, crying all the time.' 'She's doing exactly what she's supposed to be doing,' I said. The 'cheer up' mentality does not help anyone. Nor does, 'Keep yourself busy, medicate the pain, remember the good times.' If you do that, emotions get shoved underground. You can't go around it, or avoid it. You have to move into it and through it. You need to embrace the pain of the loss, lean into it."

In my own experience of losing my parents and some close friends, and certainly in my own care of patients, what Bertha says is true. It is the healthiest, but also the most challenging way to deal with grief.

"Sometimes people don't know what to say to someone who is grieving, but it's best to avoid clichés like 'time will heal,' 'be happy you had him this long,' or 'he's not suffering now.' Those stock-and-trade phrases give little comfort. Better to just be there and say nothing at all.

"If you've loved greatly, it stands to reason you are going to grieve greatly. Grief is a privilege of having loved." Bertha gives me her business card, which says, "Bringing Joy and Happiness to Others."

What would my ICU business card say, if I had one? "At Your Side During the Worst Time of Your Life" pretty much sums it up. In the hospital, we don't offer much support to grieving families, except *here's a tissue and there's the door*. Yet, some nurses and doctors have been known to attend funerals of patients, especially if they had a special bond with them. Once, a group of ICU nurses tried to organize a committee to send out condolence cards to families of people who'd died in our ICU. Some even volunteered to go out on follow-up visits to grieving families, but the project petered out. Seeing us again made them revisit a painful time. It stirred up too many unpleasant memories, and raised questions about the treatment their loved one had received. The project was a no-go.

But goodbyes are important. I remember one patient who I felt certain was going to die within the next day or two. I had spent a great deal of time speaking with her and her husband. At the end of my shift, and after my lengthy and detailed report to the nurse taking over, I was eager to hurry out of there and get home. Later that evening, before I went to bed, I realized I hadn't said goodbye to either the patient or her husband, both of whom I had connected with and whom I knew I wouldn't be seeing again. It left an uneasy feeling. I couldn't fall asleep until I phoned the ICU, asked to speak with the husband, and said goodbye. I'm glad I followed my instinct because it was, indeed, the last time I saw them.

It's been another late night. They are "working" me hard here. The wine and cheese party Suzanne arranged for me went on until midnight. These nurses sure know how to party hearty. Good thing Darin was there to drive me home.

Back at the B and B, I tiptoe up the creaky stairs so as not to disturb Twyla and her husband. "Night-night," Twyla calls out. Soon it will be dawn and she'll be up, whipping up another batch of muffins and loaves of homemade bread.

I lie in bed, wide awake, not ready for sleep, just holding the day close, mulling it over.

12

WINE AND CHEESECAKE

PEOPLE LOVE TELLING STORIES. Fishermen (and fisherwomen) boast of the big catch (or lament the one that got away); businessmen talk about closing the big deal; soldiers recount their war stories — and VON nurses recall their fondest and funniest home visits. At the gathering Suzanne hosted last night, she invited a group of nurses, both retired and actively working, who reminisced about their years visiting clients in their homes — barns, back alleys, a fleabag motel, and even a brothel. There was the younger contingent, who are still working: Nurse Manager Suzanne, Hailey, and Colleen, who was on call that night and wore a white shirt with "RN" emblazoned on it and black pants (standard nurse uniform in Nova Scotia). And then there was the old guard — Enid, Molly, Lois, and Bernadette, who wore stretch, comfy pants and colourful loose-fitting blouses, the usual uniform of women of a "certain age." As the wine flowed and a pumpkin cheesecake (Halloween is coming) was consumed, I got snapshots of the way it once was and the way it is now, one story flowing straight into another.

WHY HOME CARE?

MOLLY STARTS OFF AND TELLS IT STRAIGHT: I went into home care to get out of shift work.

COLLEEN: For years, home care *was* VON. Now, it's a business. But not in Nova Scotia. Here, it's still VON.

BERNADETTE: I started out working in the emergency department. I remember a woman who came in at change of shift with an arm fracture. Everyone was so grumpy. No one would take care of her — *you know why* — it was change of shift. That was it. I couldn't take it anymore. I'd had enough of the hospital, so I came to home care.

HAILEY: I did the opposite. I started in home care, but after a few years, I felt I needed to conquer my fear of the hospital, so I got a job there. They had all the bells and whistles but I missed the true picture of the person. And I'd forgotten about the hospital smells!

ME: I laugh whenever I call the hospital switchboard and hear the automated message: "We are a scent-free institution. . . ." Right — scent free! I'll take my chances with the nauseating Poison or migraine-inducing Opium some nurses insist on wearing. They're better than the hospital smells!

HAILEY: In the hospital, your time is never your own. If you want to spend a little extra time with a patient, you can't. The day is so regimented. Patients feel it, too. I would rather care for a person in their home than in a hospital bed, when I have to dictate what time you can do this or that or when this or that will be done to you. I cringe whenever I have to send a client to the hospital for something. I feel protective. They're not going to get the personalized care that I can provide them at home.

SUZANNE: I hated every moment working in the hospital, but I never identified what the problem was. Now I realize it was the lack of opportunity to get to know the patient and who they were other than a patient. When I got to home care, I realized that in the hospital, I couldn't be myself and I couldn't give the care I wanted to give.

ENID: I needed a change, so I decided to work for VON. Why not? They gave me a car and a bag and I could be out on the road. No doctors around. It was all up to me. In the community, patients and families place their trust in us, the nurses. They turn to us for everything. After working in the hospital for a few years, I'd had enough of the hierarchy, the rules, the regimentation. I thought, Let me out of here, I'll go work for VON.

COLLEEN: As soon as I enter a person's home, I'm in their world. Totally absorbed. I pride myself in treating everyone the same whether they have money or not. It could be a million-dollar home or a dilapidated shack that I was going into.

BERNADETTE: And sometimes you're treated better in that shack than in the mansion.

LOIS: I retired only two years ago and now I sit on the local VON board. At my job interview, I wanted the position so badly. All I could think of was if I worked in home care, I'd get to drive around town, my time would be my own, and I'd go out for lunch every day. I never ate out once. I never did. I always came back to the office, where all the nurses gathered to share our day. We became known as the lunch bunch. I enjoyed day one and the last day I worked there every bit as much. The preparation they gave me was simple: Don't sit down and don't keep narcotics in your car.

THE GOOD OLD DAYS, THE GLORY, AND THE PERKS

ENID: A VON nurse was always the first to bathe a newborn baby, even before the mother herself. Every new mother had a visit from a VON nurse when she came home from the hospital, and then at three months to see how she was doing, to make sure baby had its immunizations.

SUZANNE: My VON nurse taught me how to care for my baby when I was a new mom and gave me the confidence that I could do it.

BERNADETTE: When someone came home after surgery, they knew a VON nurse would be there. And they were. When my own mother was dying at home, I couldn't handle it alone. In walked the VON nurse with her bag and I knew all would be taken care of. And it was.

COLLEEN: Each day, I'm excited to get to work. Every day is different. My husband says I never complain about my work. I think of all the grouchy people in the hospital. Whenever I encountered a pleasant person in the hospital, it took me by surprise.

LOIS: At lunch, we were like homing devices. We got together and couldn't get enough of each other, because most days we were out there on our own. For a once-a-month treat we met at the Ranch 'n' Reef for dinner. [Nova Scotians call lunch "dinner," and what I call dinner, they call "supper." However, the question remains: What is lunch?] Nowadays, they have phone conferences, teleconferences, et cetera. But back then, we got together for meals and meetings.

MOLLY: You were a jack-of-all-trades. You had to be creative, think on your feet, figure things out yourself. Improvise. I liked that.

ENID: At my job interview, I was shaking from nerves. They asked me only two questions: "Can you draw blood?" and "Can you drive a stick shift?" Those were the requirements. To get a job with VON was a wonderful thing. I stayed until I retired. Oh, and the VON cars! The Lion's Club gave us cars. This was long before Oprah was giving away cars. They hired me to work on a Coast Guard boat. Remember that old series of Cherry Ames' stories? Well, I was Cherry Ames, Coast Guard Nurse. Cherry Ames, District Nurse. Adventures galore.

HAILEY: We have a real team spirit here. There's no gossiping, back-stabbing, or bullying. It's not part of our work culture, like it is in the hospital.

GETTING THERE IS HALF THE FUN

MOLLY: Once, to get to a diabetic in a blizzard, I had to go out on a back hoe.

BERNADETTE: "What's the house number?" I asked the husband on the phone. He sends his wife out to check. "What colour is your house?" He sends his wife back out to check the colour. Somehow, I found it.

ENID: "How far from such and such," we'd always be asking. Our first job was figuring out where to go and how to get in once you got

there. We had to be experts at finding places – long before GPS –
and figuring out the entrances because front doors aren't always
where you would think they'd be.

ME: Hospital nurses often feel stressed and overworked. Even the
newbies complain of burnout. How come I don't hear that from
any of you?

MOLLY SPEAKS FOR THEM ALL: We never looked at our work that way. If
there were challenges, we worked harder. We felt proud of our work
because we always felt we were helping people.

HOME SWEET HOME

COLLEEN: You get used to things you see. You go in some homes and
there is so much clutter, others where there's dirt. Still others
where there's both. The only thing that bothers me is bugs. In one
house I visit, there are cockroaches everywhere. I stand the whole
time I'm there.

LOIS: Every newspaper that had ever come into the house was saved.
A Christmas poinsettia left since spring. Styrofoam trays from
meat. Tools and toys, typewriters and trash. There are so many
hoarders out there – way more than we'll ever know.

BERNADETTE: One client saved every corn, callus, cuticle, and toenail
ever cut off her feet and fingers. She made a display and labelled
each from when and from which limb every item came.

MOLLY: I remember a client who was living alone in a 150-year-old
farmhouse, no plumbing, no electricity, no water, only a well, but
she was happy. I had to start a wood fire to sterilize the instruments,
even the glass syringes had to be boiled to give her insulin.

ENID: At one house, there was a big hole in the wall. I could see right
through to the next room. "See that?" the client said. "The last
nurse was doing my dressing, fell back, and bashed into the wall."
In another house, I once found a man nearly frozen to death. He
had on gumboots with holes in them and grey socks that I had to
peel off because they were stuck to his foot. He hadn't changed

them in months. I put a swipe of Vicks VapoRub under my nose to dull the stink and got to work cleaning him up. He had to go to the hospital and the stench was so bad, the ambulance guys ran out gagging and vomiting, but by then, I was used to it. I was so focused on what I was doing.

MOLLY: Sterile field? What sterile field? That's a joke. You try keeping a sterile field where a rooster is hopping around and pecking at everything. I told one lady to boil the instruments before I arrived and I would find them simmering together in a pot with boiled potatoes.

ENID: That reminds me. At one home I used to visit, there was always a pot of soup on the stove. I swear it was the same pot, the same soup, but she just kept adding things to it. One time there were feathers in it. I will never forget her; it was a sad situation. She had taken a drink from a soda can, thinking it was Coke, but it was car oil.

MOLLY: In one house there was a terrible smell, cobwebs everywhere. I fell through the wooden floor; it was rotten. The client lay in dirty, tangled sheets. He had a beard down to his waist. It took four hours to get him clean but it was so satisfying. I held my nose and got in there and bathed him. I took out the dirty mattress and got him a new one and clean linens and clothes. I had to start a fire to burn the mattress.

WHAT WE DID

ENID: A lot has changed. Our scope of practice is growing all the time. Things I used to do when I started, home care workers do now. Things doctors did in the hospital, nurses now do in the home.

SUZANNE: When central lines first came in, we felt overwhelmed. "We can't do this in people's homes," I protested. I knew it was a big undertaking. We know the safety risks of an intravenous that leads straight into the heart. Yikes — pulmonary embolus, infection, a clot, a perforation — a simple air bubble could be lethal. The nurse needs to know exactly where the line is positioned and frequently check the external length to ensure it hasn't migrated. There must be good backflow. The nurse has to ensure the line is clear and flushes easily. Resistance could indicate a clot or that the line's gotten pushed up alongside a vessel wall, or knotted or gotten kinked. It's up to the nurse, who is alone in that person's house, to keep clients safe.

ME: In the hospital, we confirm the placement of every central line with an x-ray, but obviously that's not feasible in someone's home. The crash cart and a code team are always available if needed. I can't imagine being in someone's home with a patient lying on a couch in front of the TV and something goes wrong. *Who ya gonna call? Ghostbusters!*

LOIS: I had a client whose blood sugar was 2.0. He was almost comatose. I looked in the fridge. There was only a beer so I gave him that. I found a little package of strawberry jam from Tim Hortons and I gave him that, too.

SUZANNE: I'm sorry to go on again about central lines, but they really freaked me out when we first started doing them. It's hard enough to keep them sterile in the hospital; it's been a real challenge to learn how to accomplish that in clients' homes.

ADVOCACY

HAILEY: When I went back to work in the hospital, we admitted a homeless woman one day. I washed her hair with nice shampoo, styled it, bathed her, and talked to her. The hospital nurses were taken aback at how I treated her, but it was because of being a home care nurse. When you see people in their own environment, you develop more empathy. You're less likely to judge.

COLLEEN: People have a right to say no, to refuse our care. It's not like in the hospital where it's basically "take it or there's the door." We'll still work with them. We don't give up on anybody.

MOLLY (NUDGING LOIS): That reminds me. Tell Tilda about the time you and I almost landed in jail.

LOIS (SMILING): This lady — Myrtle — had very brittle diabetes, and often went into a hypoglycemic state. So every day, Molly and I got there first thing to make her breakfast. She lived at the centre of town, so we'd meet there and plan our day together. It was our "war room." One day Molly arrived first and called me. "Lois, you better come quick." Myrtle was beside herself. The SPCA took her dog, Buster, away, because he bit an intruder, a Peeping Tom. That dog was so protective of Myrtle. When she went into the bank, Buster would wait outside and growl at anyone who went in. No one could go into the bank until Myrtle came out. I promised Myrtle we'd get Buster back, though I had no idea how I would keep that promise. The Mounties said the dog was dangerous and would have to be put down. We convinced the doctor to write a note stating that destroying the dog would be injurious to the client's mental health. We suggested that the dog's teeth be removed. Myrtle agreed. She was desperate to save her dog. The vet took out only the sharp incisors, but that was enough to get the dog released and back to Myrtle, with the stipulation that she keep him inside at all times. So, all's well that end's well — or so we thought. Not quite. In no time, Myrtle let Buster out again, roaming around, snarling at everyone as before. We were so exasperated. "Myrtle, we're going to be thrown in jail because of you." "I'll visit you," she said.

NURSE SAFETY

COLLEEN: They tell us not to go into a home if it is dangerous, that we have a right to work in a safe environment. But we'd never visit half the people we do if that was the case! [I think of Leala and her machete-wielding client.]

ENID: What about those "Beware of Dog" signs? Often they don't mean anything, but sometimes they do. At some houses, there's no sign, but there should be. Once, there was a barking, vicious dog, the kind drug dealers use to guard their stash, a Rottweiler, I think. I still went to the visit. I used my VON bag as a shield and planned to use it as a weapon, if needed. "Your dog is scary," I told the client. "You might want to think of mentioning the dog before someone comes over." Now, VON has a "no pets" policy. Clients have to put their pet away when the nurse comes.

HAILEY: Once, I was in an apartment building and the elevator door opened and a dog charged at me. Luckily, I managed to get the doors closed in time.

LOIS: Once, I was attacked by a rooster. I still have a scar. At another client's house, I couldn't leave because there was a black bear outside the front door.

ENID: Once, I went in and realized I was in a marijuana grow-op. There were weed plants everywhere. I decided to look the other way and commend his interest in horticulture.

LOIS: In one home, there was a shotgun leaning against the wall. "Is that a gun?" I asked. I was so naïve. He grabbed it and put it away. "It's just a starter pistol," he told me.

MOLLY: I didn't feel unsafe as often as you'd think – not even at the home of one sweet old lady and some shady characters. Her house was full of car parts, tools, and machinery. They belonged to her son, she told me. She told me not to visit after lunch, only in the morning. Once, I was running late, and when I arrived six men were sitting around the kitchen table that had stacks of hundred-dollar bills on it, and a few empty forty-ounce liquor bottles. Other guys were passed out on the couch. A boom box was blasting. The old lady saw me and whacked the guys in the head. "Get out! Get out! The nurse is here." A gun fell out of someone's holster. She had two dogs: one's name was Piss-Arse and the other, Motherfucker. It was a chop shop; they took parts from stolen cars and sold them for big bucks. There was a garage across the street and a mechanic asked me, "You actually went in there?" He was amazed at my bravery, but it was really naïveté. Later, I found out the old lady and the gangsters were a part of a Canada-wide drug ring.

ME: You were very dedicated.

MOLLY: Or foolish. The funny thing is, nothing bad ever happened, despite what seems like risky situations. We felt protected because we were VON nurses. Crazy, isn't it? People needed our care and so we went in.

LOIS: It's true. There was an unwritten code, that you didn't touch a VON nurse. It was a prestige we enjoyed. You had a lot of pride when you drove your VON car, and felt it gave you immunity from harm.

HAILEY: In a Halifax apartment building, straight off the elevator, I smelled ganga. Three Rastafarian families lived together in a two-bedroom apartment. I had no problem going in there. I felt safe.

BERNADETTE: It could be a bad storm, freezing temperatures, a hurricane, whatever. We went out in all conditions. Nothing stopped us. We had to get to the patient, no matter what.

PETS, LIVESTOCK, MENAGERIES

COLLEEN: Forget about dog problems - there should be a "no squirrels" policy. That's what I'm dealing with now. At a home visit the other day, my client and his wife were sitting in the middle of the kitchen floor on overturned buckets, each with a rifle, shooting at red squirrels that were scurrying along the attic beams. I swear, the two of them looked like Ma and Pa Kettle. When I changed the man's dressing, I felt a squirrel brush up against my arm.

MOLLY: One lady used to call us to treat her animals. She couldn't afford the veterinarian. She even took the animal medicine herself, like the horses' salve for a burn on her hand. She had cat food in her fridge, but little else.

LOIS: Remember the Bird Man? His house was full of pigeons – what a racket they made, and pigeon poo everywhere. A pigeon jumped on the bed while I was changing a dressing. That client lived for his birds, and who are we to try to change that?

HAILEY: I once bathed a flea-infested dog and gave insulin to the cat. You have to use a 25 gauge, but still get down into the subcutaneous tissues. If you just go too superficially, under the fur, it doesn't get absorbed properly.

ME: Good to know.

ENID: Does anyone remember the house with the horse in the living room? A new bylaw stated you couldn't keep a horse in the city so they hid him in the house. I was changing a dressing when all of a sudden, I hear a neigh. "What is that?" I asked, though it was unmistakably a horse.

LOIS: A cat peed in my bag once.

BERNADETTE: Dogs? Dogs are nothing compared to Susie the Monkey. Her owner ran a boarding house [air quotes]. It was really a brothel. Susie, the spider monkey, sat on her shoulder and threw her poos at anyone who came near. I'll never forget walking past her cage and her screeching at me, her arms clawing at me through the bars as I walked down a long, dark hall.

THERE'S NO PLACE LIKE HOME

SUZANNE: Even if a client chooses to live in unsafe conditions, we have to respect their choices. I recall a morbidly obese patient – over five hundred pounds – who lived in her bed. She couldn't have gotten out in an emergency. She was trapped in her body and trapped in her home. She left the door unlocked, because she couldn't get up to let me in. She was also a hoarder and had no money, so her possessions were trash and garbage she'd collected.

HAILEY: I've been in houses that have been condemned, but as my dad used to say, you never know what another person is going through. He made us clean toilets and give rides to these local mentally handicapped people. He wanted to keep us humble.

SUZANNE: VON nurses taught me about respect. I had to learn that "normal" is not how I define it. People have a right to live the way they want to live.

DYING AT HOME

MOLLY: I was always hyperactive, and palliative care calmed me
down. You have to slow down when you're caring for dying
patients. I loved palliative care and did it almost exclusively in the
last six years until retirement. Some of my best moments as a nurse
were bringing comfort and dignity to people in their final days.
I'll never forget a young mother with sarcoma. She wanted to die
at home, but toward the end, she went into respiratory distress and
we decided to take her to the hospital. She said, "Wait. I have to
make my bed first." Then she went to the hospital to die. Another
client, a man in his eighties, was in congestive heart failure. I visited
him in his trailer and stayed with him until the end. But I had no
meds to offer him. That was a painful death for him – for me, too.
I'll never forget it. Lois helped change all of that. You tell what
happened, Lois dear.

LOIS: I cared for a patient who died in excruciating pain. The doctor
wouldn't order anything without seeing him. He told me to bring
him to the hospital, but the patient was too uncomfortable and
unstable to move – I didn't want him to die on the way. Easy for the
doctor – he wasn't there to hear the patient's cries, or look him in
the eyes and tell him, "I have nothing to relieve your pain." I'll
never forget the family's eyes, begging me to give him something
to relieve his pain, and their fury at me when I had nothing to offer.
A few days later, at a team meeting, Molly nudged me to tell them
what happened. But I was shy; I couldn't speak to doctors. What if
they felt I was criticizing them or overstepping their territory? But
I found the courage and got up to speak. I tried to control my emotions, but there were tears in my eyes.

SUZANNE: Lois's speaking up was the impetus to develop the Symptom
Relief Kit. There's no need to admit people to hospital for pain control. If they truly want to die at home, pain management – and all
other symptoms of dying – can be accomplished.

SUZANNE: Before we had the Symptom Relief Kit, patients were dying agonizing deaths at home or were transferred to the hospital to die on a stretcher in the emergency room. After Lois spoke up about her experience, it pushed us to develop a Symptom Relief Kit that contains meds for the common discomforts of the dying process: anxiety, secretions, nausea, pain, seizures. We taught the families how to administer the drugs if a nurse wasn't there. This innovation has allowed people to die at home in comfort. Of course, there are risks with lay people administering drugs, and having narcotics out in the community. In one instance, we discovered that a son was selling his mother's Dilaudid on the streets, depriving her of pain meds. But in most cases, it works out just fine. Now, nurses are allowed to pronounce a death. They do not need to wait for the doctor to arrive or, worse, have to transfer a client to the hospital so an ECG can be done to prove the obvious with a documented flat line.

BERNADETTE (CHUCKLING): When I worked in the ER and they'd bring in a cold corpse just so we could document the death, I'd make it show a reading by jiggling the bed a little, just to freak them out.

ENID: Remember the eccentric doctor who'd fall asleep while you'd be talking to him, especially over the phone? He'd write his orders on a napkin or on the back of an envelope or any scrap of paper. He had a thing about enemas. Once, I called to tell him a patient had died. "Give him a soapsuds enema. That'll revive him." "I can do that, doctor, but he'll still be dead," I said.

UNUSUAL REQUESTS

HAILEY: A client asked me to meet him in his barn. "My cow is sick," he said. At his request, I took its temperature, but had no idea what was normal for a cow.

LOIS: Speaking of cows – that reminds me – I once had to milk a cow for a client. This cow wasn't partial to strangers and she let me know her displeasure. Let's just say I had to go home to change my clothes and take a shower.

BERNADETTE: I cut the hair of a black woman and it stuck out, making her look like a porcupine. What to do? I went to the drugstore to buy special gel to tame it down before her son got home.

COLLEEN: Just the other day, a client told me how much he could get for me if I performed certain services on the street.

ME (GASPING): What did you say?

COLLEEN: "You couldn't afford me!"

LOIS: Once, I changed the clothes on a corpse when the family didn't like what she was wearing.

BERNADETTE: One night I got a call late at night. "I need you to come. My penis pains." So, I had to go out in the middle of the night to change a crotchety old man's catheter.

ENID: I used to keep a pile of newspaper in the back of the car to rest my bag on it, if the house was too dirty.

BERNADETTE: One woman kept a dead cat at the end of her bed. She didn't believe it was dead, so wouldn't let me dispose of it for her.

CLIENT APPRECIATION

HAILEY: I was given a toaster, once. Another time, a lobster. A live one. And every Christmas an elderly client tried to give me a tip. I tried to explain why I could not accept money. One year, I thought I had gotten through to her when all I received was a wrapped box of Pot of Gold chocolates. I always gave the garbage men Christmas gifts. This one busy year, my children began to holler as the truck rolled up the street on the last pick-up day before Christmas. I had forgotten to buy them something, so I grabbed the box from Mrs. P and ran outside. The truck lingered, then blew the horn, and the two men waved at me. I felt warm inside that they appreciated my gift. Later, my boss asked if I'd opened the present. She said Mrs. P had put a twenty-dollar bill on top of the box.

LOIS: Back in the eighties, we had to collect payment for each visit. An elderly man I saw weekly for a bath paid two dollars for a visit. One day he told me wanted to give me a raise – to $2.25.

MOLLY: Years ago, in the Annapolis Valley, I cared for an AIDS patient. His partner had died and he had to move in with his elderly parents due to his failing health. The farming community and friends shunned him. His father never accepted his sexuality. I cared for him until he died at home. His funeral was by invitation only and I was invited. What an honour.

The next morning on the drive from Yarmouth to Halifax, I scan the horizon for Oreo cows, red squirrels, and spider monkeys. Don't spot any, so I drop off for a snooze. I loved last night, where I enjoyed wine but no whine. None of the griping or whinging, none of the put-upon, hard-done-by, I-don't-get-no-respect, they-don't-pay-us-what-we're-worth attitude that too many hospital nurses have. That probably doesn't describe the majority of us, but one could easily get that impression, as those nurses are the most vocal and noisy. When hospital nurses get together, it seems like there's always something to gripe about or to feel indignant, even outraged, about. Complaining feels so good – getting it off your chest, discharging your bile, shooting off your mouth – but it leaves an unpleasant aftertaste.

I open a paper I'd folded and put into my purse. Last night, as I was leaving, Lois gave me a photocopy of a newspaper article written by Nurse Letty Neaves Drennan, a graduate of the local school of nursing, class of 1946, who became a member of the Victorian Order of Nurses. She describes the "techniques for a proper home visit."

When you arrived at the home, if it was a new case or your first time there, you introduced yourself and asked if they had a section of newspaper. You unzipped your sleeves and folded them up, took the green soap and a paper towel to the bathroom sink, and washed your hands using the paper bag for your used towel.

At this point, you attached your white cotton apron with its button hole at the top onto the second brass button on your uniform jacket and tied the apron ties. For whatever care you had to give, you took what you required and sat it on the newspaper, closed the bag and you started the care and didn't open it again unless you washed your hands.

. . . I recall one home I went to where the young boy who was a little backward had had an operation and I was visiting to do his dressing. The mother's love for him was so evident and she was coaching him in such a way in social graces and behavior that I am sure he achieved his potential and more. I can still feel that love between the mother and her son.

In these fast-paced times of constant change and with the world in flux, it is comforting to know some things are immutable, timeless. It's just like Stuart McLean, Canada's foremost storyteller, writes in his book, *Notes from the Neighbourhood*, "*Everything* changes and then – *nothing* changes."

13

THE SMILING GOAT

JUSTIN DEFTLY JUGGLES MULTIPLE BALLS. They're his morning clients we're going to visit in downtown Halifax, all within walking distance. One wants to be seen first thing in the morning; two others live in the same building, but one wants him to come in the morning, the other in the afternoon, after she's had her hair done.

"No worries. I'll swing back later," he tells her cheerfully.

In the hospital it's more like, *I'm here. It's now. Now or never. Take it or leave it. You, your family, your meds, your pain, your needs – they're on my schedule.*

Just when I thought I'd seen all there was to see in home care, I get to accompany Nurse Justin Bragg on his rounds. It doesn't take me long to realize that Justin has a few things to teach me. He parks his car on a tree-lined boulevard that leads in one direction to Dalhousie University and in the other to the city centre. From here, we'll go on foot, client to client. Before we enter each home, Justin gives me a brief summary of each client's history.

We see Wanda first. She's a retired pediatrician living on her own in a downtown apartment building. When Justin first started taking care of her a year ago, she enjoyed peppering Justin with questions to test his medical knowledge. Lately, her mental condition has been declining. Wanda had always been a meticulous dresser and well groomed, but a few days ago, Justin came in to find her standing in the kitchen with her bra on backwards, her hair askew. Today, Wanda looks forlorn. Her housecoat is rumpled and dirty, and it doesn't take a stretch of the imagination to envision one of her droopy sleeves getting snagged on a stove burner.

Last night, Wanda had a fever and went to the ER, where she was diagnosed with a urinary tract infection and sent home. "I'm feeling better today, Sylvia," she tells Justin. "I don't need those pills anymore."

Justin doesn't correct the name she calls him, nor when she asks me, looking over at him adoringly, "Don't you just love the women of VON?"

"Yes, Justin is a fine woman," I say, teasing him and going along with her mix-up.

Justin takes her temp — at 37.8°C it's elevated — and asks if she's tired. "Yes, from wasting my time last night in the hospital. I demand that something constructive be done right away." Justin gently explains that she has a fever and must continue to take the antibiotics until they're finished. He tells her that a storm is brewing and Hurricane Sandy is on its way. It might hit Halifax, so Justin suggests backup plans in case the storm prevents him from getting to her, but she isn't listening. She's staring at the pills he's offering her.

"Are these mine?" Her eyes narrow at him. "They're not my pills." He checks each bottle together with her, but she's still not ready to take them. "They're not the right colour. Are you giving me the *genetic* pills or the real ones?"

As a doctor, I'm quite sure she knew the difference between generic and trade medications — could probably even describe their molecular composition. Justin brings her a glass of water to take her pills. "I make them laugh, I make them cry," she mutters and drinks them down. Justin sits at her dining room table, finishing up his charting. He nods at that and also when she says, "You'll never know what you'll find in these boxes down there." She searches under the table, then looks up to tell us about a tasty lunch she ate years ago. "It was the best turkey sandwich. It didn't need mayonnaise. It was a wild turkey brought up in the field."

"A happy turkey," Justin says, again joining her where she is.

"How much longer can Wanda live on her own?" I ask Justin as we walk along the sidewalk to the next client. "She's right on the edge."

"It's a fine line, isn't it? She wants her independence, but at what point does it affect her safety? Does she have a right to live in a way that is unsafe? She lives in an apartment building, so her actions could affect other people. Is she mentally competent enough to make that choice? Some days yes, some days no. In the elderly, an infection almost always compromises their mental status, so her confusion may be transient. There are many factors that need to be taken into consideration. It's complicated."

"So, what do you do, so that you can sleep at night – so that we all can?"

"Today, there's a significant change in Wanda's state of mind. I'll call the office and arrange for another nurse to visit this evening and we'll take it from there and monitor her closely. The goal with Wanda is her goal – to keep her home as long as possible."

The consensus is clear, but only now do I fully realize it: everyone wants to be home.

We go up the elevator of an apartment building to meet Maude, who is morbidly obese to the point of near immobility. She is a diabetic who complains of pains in her legs. Justin examines them and finds nothing of concern. "You've got to keep moving," he encourages her.

"I'm perfectly okay," she tells me as Justin takes her blood pressure. "As long as I can stay at home."

Maude's doctor has made adjustments in her medications, but the new meds haven't been delivered yet from the pharmacy. "I'll check with you later to make sure you got them. Your blood pressure is a little high today." I have a feeling that call is also intended to be a reminder for her to actually take them. These pills can't be skipped. Her blood pressure is high at 170 over 100. Justin is all over this minutia. These small things are huge; each detail could be a matter of life or death, just like in the ICU, come to think of it.

"How's the blood sugar?" Justin asks.

"Oh, it's right as rain," she tells him, and shows him her daily recordings. "I have diabetes. But just a little bit, mind you."

"Your numbers are good," Justin says, and she beams. "I'll do anything so that I can stay at home," she says again. "I need a little help now and then, but I'm seventy-five and when you get old, people wait on you."

"You deserve it," I say.

Maude looks at Justin. "I don't know what I would do without Justin."

Fortunately, Maude also has ample family supports, friends that check up on her daily, and neighbours that run errands for her. It's an ideal arrangement. But a disruption in any component of this set-up — a break in the chain or a loose link — could threaten the whole system. These fragile elders living alone in the community are teetering on the brink between life and death.

One thing is obvious: Justin is loved by all. For some clients, his visit is clearly the highlight of their day. They await his arrival and all have questions ready for him: How should I handle . . . ? What should I do if . . . ? Why does . . . ? If my rash looks worse . . . ."

There's another common feature with all of Justin's clients. In each home, the kitchen table is command central; it's the "headquarters" for treasured items, equipment, supplies, and sometimes random objects.

On Wanda's kitchen table there was a jar of leaky batteries, a huge magnifying glass, a stack of dated Hungarian newspapers, and old photographs.

On Maude's table there was a plastic toothpick dispenser; a serviette holder; a basket full of pill bottles; silk flowers in a vase; a mug of dried-up pens; a bottle of hardened coral-coloured nail polish; lion, elephant, and monkey letter openers; salt and pepper shakers (salt is Santa and pepper is Rudolph the Red-Nosed Reindeer); an automatic blood pressure cuff still in its unopened box from the store; and a mini tower of sugar-free cookies.

Saskia is our next client, and while Justin attends to her, I cop a glance into her kitchen: on the table is a stained quilted placemat, a Barbie doll stuck into a toilet roll holder, a ceramic duck with a blue ribbon around its neck, a pile of cassette tapes of Russian folk songs, a jar of pennies, and a handwritten list of phone and PIN numbers.

Since Saskia is on an antibiotic and Coumadin, a blood thinner, which may interact, Justin calls the lab to arrange for a blood test to check if she needs a medication adjustment. Then he calls her son, Boris, to remind him to make sure she gets the blood test. Fortunately, he's able to take time off work to get that done.

"My son is in charge of me," Saskia says proudly. "He takes care of all my affairs."

I consider that disclosure. Even in some of the "best" families, there's always potential for financial shenanigans, but what choice does a vulnerable elder like Saskia have?

Saskia has talked with Justin about moving in with Boris and his family, or possibly going to an assisted living home, and, one day, a nursing home.

"Be good to your kids," she advises me. "If you're not, don't expect they'll be good to you."

She and I chat while Justin puts in a call to the pharmacist to alert him to a possible change in Saskia's Coumadin prescription, and to get her pills administered in a blister pack, which will make it easier for her to take the right ones at the right time. He knows she can be a little confused at times. In fact, as we are chatting, she gets up suddenly, goes to the kitchen, and stands there looking puzzled. She opens a cupboard door, then shuts it. Opens a drawer, then slides it closed again. "I can't remember what I came here for." Standing there looking puzzled, she takes a sip of her now-cold coffee.

We leave her to figure that out and Justin adds her to the list of clients who now need to be seen by a nurse twice daily. Justin's next client is Marnie, whose messy apartment is full of souvenirs from around the world — African masks and pre-Columbian figurines, Persian rugs, and Greek archeological finds. Despite these beautiful things, when I peek into her kitchen, there is no table at all.

Marnie is — or once was — stunning. Her classic beauty has been ravaged by alcoholism. A photograph of her smiling, standing with a pilot beside an old DC-47, shows she was once statuesque, with wavy auburn hair and a great figure. Now, she's thin and sad-looking. As unscientific as this sounds, she looks *unwell*. Her hair is unwashed and her faded cotton shirt is wrinkled and buttoned on the wrong holes.

"Applesauce," she says listlessly, when Justin asks what she ate for breakfast.

A string quartet plays on a dusty old turntable. I concentrate on the music to avoid thinking about Marnie. It's Beethoven's *String Quartet, No. 14*. Cerebral and ethereal, it's one of his last compositions before he died, a piece of music that has fond associations for me of an old boyfriend, a music major, who taught me a lot — about music, that is. (Not Mr. Thunder Bay of the "New York was taken" line, another beau.) For a few moments, it takes me away.

Before we arrived, Justin had told me he stays alert for signs she's drinking again. One morning, a few weeks ago, she came to the door stark naked, and slurring her speech. At first he thought she was having a stroke but then realized she was drunk.

"How's the drinking, Marnie?" he asks gently.

"Haven't had a drop for awhile. Six days."

"Good girl," he says in an encouraging, but not patronizing, way.

"But what did you actually do there, for Marnie?" I wonder out loud as Justin and I walk along a downtown street with funky little boutiques and cafés on either side. "It was like a social visit. How can that be cost-effective?"

"My purpose was to check on her. That helps her stay at home. It costs our health care system fifty-five dollars for my visit, which is a lot less than if she was in a nursing home."

We stop at The Smiling Goat, a hip little coffee shop next to the elegant Lord Nelson Hotel and take a break to sip espressos and talk about – what else? – wounds. Typical nurse convo. Incredibly, there are a lot of people walking around with breaks in their skin and holes in their bodies. There are necrotic gangrenous wounds, diabetic amputations, dehiscence when a wound ruptures, pilonidal cysts (deep, painful fissures, often around the rectum, that require packing), ragged venous stasis wounds, and cookie-cutter arterial wounds. (In the hospital I have seen extreme wounds. Recently, we had a patient from a nursing home who was admitted to the ICU with sepsis from a nasty pressure ulcer wound on his buttocks. Privately, we called it the "swimming pool," because it was fluid-filled, had a deep end and a shallow end, and a flap of skin that looked like a diving board (maybe "you had to be there . . .").) We chatter about malodorous drainage, serous ooze, and purulent pus while we drink delicious coffee. Justin is an expert in wound care, but if he encounters a tricky or unusual wound, or something he's unfamiliar with, he snaps a photograph and sends it to a wound care nurse specialist for a consultation.

As we walk along the boulevard, Justin talks on the phone to a public health nurse about the safety of giving two live immunizations at the same time. He's going to see a child this afternoon who needs her vaccines. "Yes . . . okay, so it's safe to give two live viruses on the same day," he says over the roar of the passing traffic. "But if I give only one, I have to give the second a month later." He gets off the phone. "In the community, you've got to communicate with others – doctors, pharmacists, social workers, whoever has the information you need."

"It should be like that in the hospital, too, but we're not always team players."

We walk a few blocks to the apartment building of the next client and, since the door is open, we walk right in. Instantly, I'm in shock. Justin forgot to prepare me for the sight before my eyes. From the door to the walls, from floor to ceiling, on all the walls, in every space and crevice, upon every surface, there's *stuff*. Lucy, his client, calls

out to us from where she lies in her bedroom, on her bed in the midst
of more stuff. Her bed is so loaded up there's only a narrow strip
for her to sleep. (As for the kitchen table, there's neither a kitchen
nor a table.)

Justin and I wade and weave through a tangle of electrical cords and
TV cables and scattered hillocks of clothes to get to her. With each step,
it's impossible not to tread on something. Lucy's bedroom is dark with
the curtains drawn, and the bed is so overloaded with objects that I
have to look twice to make out Lucy herself. She's a thin, wispy woman
in her fifties and has numerous oozing ulcers all over her body; to me,
it looks like she's scratched herself and made sores that have become
infected. They are so painfully sensitive that even the edges of the
gauze press and chafe.

"Don't fold the bandages," she barks at Justin. "They feel like tour-
niquets. I want to rip them off. Last night, I was ready to take a scissors
to your hard work."

While Justin does his work, Lucy watches *Say Yes to the Dress* on the
TV. A bride gazes at herself in the mirror and appraises what she sees
with hopeful eyes. Her tummy bulges and breasts spill out over the top.
"I'm not sure this dress is for me," she says.

"I assure you, it's not, you idiot," Lucy says, with a snort of derision.

Luckily, she has her TV show to distract her somewhat, because the
dressing change is tedious and uncomfortable. Then Justin has to start
a new IV in her arm, which she finds most disagreeable, too. Justin
runs an antibiotic into the new line, and chats with Lucy.

As we wait for the IV infusion to finish, I can't take my eyes off a
jumble of Christmas decorations (china angels that meld into faded
wreaths, scented candles in dusty glasses, a blow-up Santa doll,
unopened bags of potpourri, rolls of gift wrap), jars of springs, screws,
and keys, ancient TV converters, stacks of wire hangers, a pile of plastic purses, a rusted bird cage, a tennis racquet missing strings with TV
bunny ears poking through it. There's nowhere to sit, so I stand outside her bedroom door and gaze at a mountain of hats, bags full of bags,

mounds of wrinkled clothes, scattered piles of compact discs and VHS tapes, a laundry basket full of old shoes, a Donald Duck plush toy . . .

There's so much to look at! Clear Rubbermaid tubs filled with ribbons, string, and acrylic paint bottles; strewn fabric swatches; a typewriter on the floor, keys missing and a spool of ribbon unravelling out of it; a beat-up red-and-white striped, circus-type popcorn maker whose popping days are long gone; a colourful swirl of scarves; a bundle of empty toilet paper rolls; and a lineup of empty Mason jars with no lids . . . I peel my eyes away, if only to give them a rest from this visual onslaught.

Lucy had a urinary catheter and frequent bladder infections, which have led to a problem with incontinence. Justin reminds her about the exercises he's taught her to retrain her bladder. Though she loves coffee, it exacerbates her condition, but Justin promises to bring her one, as a treat – from the Smiling Goat, of course – on his next visit.

I have to wonder: given the fact that Lucy has poor balance, limited mobility, almost no movement in her legs, and weakness in her arms and hands, what are the logistics of collecting and storing such a stash? I'm just being pragmatic. How does she scavenge and dumpster dive from a wheelchair? That could really impair your ability to carry out your compulsions. How do you get your fix for this addiction? Do you have to enlist help? I can feel how this stuff – what most would charitably refer to as "junk" – is companionship and comfort to Lucy. Perhaps she's attached to these things like others are attached to their family or to their pets.

Justin is not the only one caring for Lucy. An occupational therapist visits and works to help her part with items, one at a time. A physical therapist assists her to strengthen her upper body for using the wheelchair. A speech language therapist helps her speak more audibly and clearly. A public guardian handles her money because Lucy is a compulsive shopper and would blow through it all and be broke in no time.

Back in Justin's car he does his charting and makes a few phone calls. I keep quiet to allow him to concentrate, but after a few minutes, he looks up from his notes, looks out the windshield, and says simply, "I love home care."

"I feel that way about the ICU."

"Here's what I like about home care. The independence. Relying on yourself. Personalizing care to each individual. Using all of your skills. Our scope of practice is expanding all the time. What RNs used to do now we do."

(Long ago on this journey, I abandoned the prejudice against practical nurses that a lot of hospital nurses still harbour. To them, only RNs are real nurses. To them, I say, meet Justin Bragg, a registered practical nurse and a real nurse by anyone's standards.)

"Another thing is that out here in the community, everyone inside the client's circle of care works with each other. There's true collaboration, real teamwork."

"In the hospital, there are still hierarchies, and we're not great at collaborating with other services and departments. Sometimes the right hand doesn't know what the left is doing."

Something else occurs to me, and though it's a weird observation, I go ahead and ask anyway. "I'm curious, Justin. Was it just a coincidence that all your clients today were female?"

"Yes, just a coincidence," he says, "but with one slight exception. There are times when Lucy is 'Eddie,' an eight-year-old boy, and he's very mischievous, always getting in trouble at school." In addition to Eddie, Lucy has three more distinct people inside herself, each with their own personalities, behaviours, likes and dislikes. Justin knows them all and interacts with each one as they make their appearance. "I know I'm speaking to Eddie when Lucy refers to her pills as 'my treats for being a good boy,' calls an outing 'recess,' or when she stays indoors on a rainy day and calls it 'a time-out for being a bad boy.' Another of her personalities comes out only in the third person. 'She's scared,' Lucy will say. This personality – Loretta – is the one that will express what scares Lucy."

Wow, Justin knows his clients well – all of them.

"Oh, and something else I just thought of," Justin says, still answering my question. "You're right, the clients today were all women, but Marnie was born male. She still has a penis and testicles, but she's been out for many years as a woman and dresses as one. She even managed to pass as a woman back in the day, during her stewardess years, when there was a lot of pressure to be attractive to men and keep the pilots happy."

Occasionally, for different reasons, female hospital patients request to have no male nurses assigned to their care. I think they'd feel differently if they met Justin. Justin is the nurse anyone – no, *everyone* – would want.

Tomorrow morning, I fly home. I need to get back, regroup, become reacquainted with my husband and family, and do a few shifts in the ICU so I don't lose my job. I don't know how Judith juggles so many different things – running VON, leading the nursing profession, and tirelessly traversing the world on behalf of global health. Her stamina is incredible; she's indefatigable. I'm exhausted after these few stops and can't wait to get home. I crash in my room at my lovely hotel, which is situated on the deliciously named Chocolate Lake. The employees all have nicknames like Snickers, Kit-Kat, and Twix. The hotel mascot is Cocoa, a chocolate lab, of course, who's snoozing in the lobby, stretched out in front of the fireplace. He belongs to everyone. The hotel staff take turns walking him around the lake and taking him home for the night. Cocoa is a communal dog; they share his care.

14

MOTHER OF MOTHERS

"IT'S YOUR CHOICE. *La langue de votre choix*," it says on the airport welcome sign.

It's true. *C'est vrai.*

I've quickly discovered you can greet anyone here with either "hello" or "*bonjour.*" And while Quebec is French and the rest of Canada is English, from what I can tell, New Brunswick is truly bilingual. Anyone here takes your lead and carries on in either language. And right off the plane, the people here are warm and welcoming.

So, where am I now? Moncton, New Brunswick, population 110,000. What a blast this is, touring the country on VON's tab. But I'm here on business, I remind myself, to meet teen moms and their babies. Nurse Educator Maria DesRoches has arranged a meeting in the office with Chantal, the mother of six-year-old Mimi, who sits quietly beside her on a couch, ping-ponging between colouring with crayons and playing a video game on her mother's phone. Chantal's wavy chestnut hair, parted down the centre, is like a curtain drawn to either side to reveal her dark eyes and gentle face — a look mirrored in a smaller replica by her daughter.

Mimi was a newborn and Chantal only seventeen when she was

miserably married to a World of Warcraft–gamer husband for whom the virtual world was better than the real one.

"I tried to get into it, too," Chantal recalls, "I even created my own avatar, but he pushed me away. Financially, it was tough. He sold my engagement ring. He didn't work, but at seven exactly, supper had to be on the table. Then he'd be on the computer until two or three in the morning. He didn't even care about the baby's first kick. He never showed interest in her."

Mimi interrupts her mom politely to ask for a snack and squeals with delight at what she finds in Mom's purse. "*Les poisson d'or! Les poisson d'or!*" Noticing me, she translates for my benefit, "Goldfish!" She shows me a picture of her dog on the phone. "*Il s'appelle Pitou* and he ran into *moi* and *il fait du boo boo.*" She points to a sore knee. "Sometimes I *manqué* just in time."

Chantal picks up her story. "Fortunately, I found Rock & Talk. It's a support group for teen moms. It's where I met Maria." Chantal smiles at Maria gratefully. "We talked about making a budget, getting back in shape, dealing with stress, nutrition, and our relationships. My mom told me my life was over by having a baby and dropping out of high school. She said she wouldn't support me if I was going to throw my life away. Maria became my second mom during that time. It was a bad time." Chantal covers her face and Mimi jumps up from the couch to put her arm around her. Chantal wipes her eyes and continues. "Meeting other girls with similar problems helped me, but it was a terrible time. I was not in a good place. One day this other girl was speaking about her bad situation – Maria called it psycho-logical abuse – and I realized that's what it was for me, too. He wouldn't let me out of the house, told me I was fat and ugly and I'd always be alone if I left him, no one else would want me. He said he'd get custody of Mimi because I was a bad mother. One day he was furi-ous about how I'd parked the car. I went out to move it but he got in before me and tried to run me over. Mimi was crying but he wouldn't let me go to her. That was it. 'I need to get out,' I told my parents. They

came over one day when he was at work. I was so scared I was sick –
dizzy, throwing up, headache. We packed my things. I left him a note.
Told him the truth, with a bit of water added to the wine."

At the same moment, Maria and I look over to see how Mimi is reacting. She appears to be totally engrossed in the video game, her imperious little index finger commanding a rocket to fly into outer space.
I have no doubt she is listening. Chantal realizes what we're thinking.

"I don't hide anything from Mimi. She's seen everything. There are
no secrets between us. Once, he – her father – grabbed me by the
throat and she was right there. Another time –" she stops short. She
doesn't want to talk about that time.

Chantal went back to finish high school and then applied to college
to study to become a laboratory technologist. She worked at Tim
Hortons, in a grocery store, as a waitress and a dog walker, and at a
retirement home. Her mother eventually became more supportive
and helped with babysitting. Chantal was a diligent student until a setback at school that first year.

"I wrote an exam. I was so nervous that as soon as I got into the
exam room, in pencil, I jotted down the order of the tubes for drawing
blood, you know, blue, red, green, lavender, EDTA, heparinized – on
the desk top. I got 98 per cent on the exam but the next day, I got a call
from the dean. He accused me of cheating. *Incroyable*, I thought.
'What are you talking about?' He showed me a picture of my writing
on the desk. It was an honest mistake, but they took away my 98 and
gave me a 51, so I'd pass, but just barely. It made me want to quit college and I almost did, but . . . " She looks at Maria, to show what made
her stay. "I decided I'd show them. On my next exam, I got 100 per
cent, actually 102 per cent with the bonus questions. The next year, I
made the honour roll, with perfect attendance."

Life is good now. Chantal credits her success to the Rock & Talk
group and Maria's support. "She taught me how to be a mother. I didn't
have a clue how to take care of a baby, or that you even needed a car
seat. I was so down after I had Mimi. Here was this beautiful thing, but

I felt no love for her. Luckily, in time, it came. Now, I'm a peer support to other teen moms."

"When we see someone like Chantal, who has many strengths, we knew it would help her to help others," Maria says. "We hired her for a few hours a week to help run the program."

"I've received so much. Now, it's my turn to help others." She gathers up Mimi and her toys and is about to leave when she stops and turns back. She wants to tell me what happened, the other time. "It happened a few months ago." She starts tentatively. "I was buying my house and I had to meet with him to get my name off the old house we had together. He wasn't making payments and it was giving me a bad credit rating. He had remarried and his wife was nine months' pregnant. She was cowering in the corner and looked just like me when I lived with him. Mimi was petrified, sobbing hysterically. He came up to my face to show me who's boss, but I stood up to him. 'You got another girl pregnant, but you ain't no father.' He shoved me up against the wall. I hit him with my purse. Then I had a panic attack. I was taken to the hospital. They gave me three shots of Ativan." She pounds her fist into her leg, one arm, then the other. "Boom, boom, boom." When I told the nurses what happened, they called the cops, but they didn't press charges because there were no marks on me. There was no evidence and because I had swung my purse at him, they said I'd started the altercation. So they opened a file on me!"

Chantal now has a full-time job with the Red Cross as a phlebotomist. Recently, she met a man online and they're Skype-dating. "Sometimes it's easier to talk to strangers than people you know, but for now, I'm by myself. People think I'm the nanny because there's no ring on my finger. Beyoncé is right – if he likes it, he's gotta put a ring on it – but even though I'm a single mom, I feel proud."

To get to the next stop in my itinerary, Maria drives us an hour north of Moncton along the scenic Northumberland Strait to the quaint little village of Bouctouche. I see town names along the way, like Shediac and Miramichi, that come from the Mi'kmaq First Nations people.

It's easy to talk with Maria. There's a calm openness about her that puts one at ease and makes you feel as if she has all the time in the world to discuss whatever's on your mind. She's like a beatific Madonna with her graceful hands, kind, soulful eyes, and serene demeanour. Yet, she's also a petite firebrand who knows who she is and confidently rocks a chic look in silk harem pants, a billowy paisley blouse, and open-toed shoes showing pink toenails.

Her title may be "nurse educator," but what Maria is is a professional nurturer, a mother who mothers mothers, a parent who parents parents. *Apparently.* (I couldn't resist.)

"Nurturing? Yes, I am, *bien sûr,* but I also give the firm message that these girls have to step up and get their act together for the new life they've brought into the world."

In a church basement, we attend a session of Bosom Buddies, where mothers are blissfully breast-feeding their little ones. Annik's first baby, petite Manon, was premature, at twenty-five weeks, and weighed just under two pounds. "I went from 'I hope I can breast-feed' to 'I hope my baby survives.' Manon was so weak I had to teach her how to suck. I pumped and pumped and she had only my milk," Annik says. "Then I developed mastitis. The pain was unbelievable. I would scream, but still, I breast-fed her." She was paired with a mom who'd been through similar difficulties, and who offered telephone supports and home visits.

"Mothers helping mothers is not a new invention. It's the way it always used to be," Maria says, "only now it has to be organized, because it doesn't happen naturally among the women of a village." She tells me about an annual event she helps organize where the school gymnasium is filled with breast-feeding mothers. "It's become as popular as a basketball game."

When I was at home, breast-feeding each of my two sons, I once calculated that, time- and energy-wise, it amounted to the equivalent of a full-time job with mandatory overtime. For me, it wasn't exactly a blissful experience, at least not at first, but I had a lot of support from girlfriends, and that kept me going. Had I been isolated or alone, I doubt I'd have stuck with it. I know the value of these groups.

In the early evening, in a cooking class kitchen over a no-frills grocery store, ten teen moms-to-be cluster around, buzzing with excitement. Dressed in baggy sweatpants, hoodies, and running shoes, they compare bellies and chatter about pregnancy symptoms and upcoming baby showers. I hope they'll be this happy when the baby arrives and reality hits. One girl has come to the class with her mother. Two dads have come. They sit together, slouching in their chairs, trying to be invisible, looking like they wish they were somewhere else, anywhere but here.

Maria asks questions to get a discussion going. "How much time have you spent thinking about the baby's room? Whether it will be a boy or a girl? What about baby names?"

They chatter excitedly, smiling and animated about these topics. However, at Maria's next questions, their mood becomes subdued and they fall silent.

"How much time have you spent thinking about your baby's brain development? About the kind of parent you want to be? What would you like people to say about your child when they are sixteen or seventeen, the age you are now?"

She hands out stationery for them to compose a letter to their eighteen-year-old child. "You are not just about to be parents but teachers, too."

One girl reads her letter about how hard this experience has been. Another warns her grown-up child not to do as she's done. They all write their wish that their grown-up babies will be successful and happy.

During the break, I ask Maria about labour and delivery. As I recall, those were the main topics covered in the prenatal classes my husband and I attended when I was pregnant the first time around.

"It's a luxury I can't afford. I have this one, brief window of opportunity to impress upon them the importance of the role they're about to take on."

Next, they pull topics out of a hat.

On spanking: "What is the message you're sending? That hitting is okay? Be sneaky and don't get caught? Think about what you want to teach your child. This is a blank slate, your chance to create something good."

On the topic of temper tantrums, one father has a strong opinion. "They happen because the baby is spoiled, given everything it wants." He folds his arms across his chest like that's that.

"You will not spoil a baby by responding to its needs," Maria tells them. "With a child, you must set limits, but with a baby, *pas possible*, you cannot spoil. Show up and look into the baby's eyes. The message you want to give whenever your baby cries is, *Hello. I'm here.* If you don't show up each time, there will be a loss of trust."

She tries to impress upon the fathers that their role is more than doing chores and paying for things. She advises them not to yell, and to walk away when stressed until they calm down.

"What reaction did you get from your parents when you told them about your pregnancy?" she asks the class.

"No one said congratulations."

"I got thrown out of the house."

"My parents couldn't believe how stupid I was."

"My mother told me I'd ruined my life. She asked me, 'Are you trying to kill yourself?'"

"Maria was the first person who congratulated me."

After the class, I sit with Maria and tell her I was surprised to hear she'd congratulated the teen moms. "It sounds as if you approve of the situation they're in. They have such a hard road ahead of them."

Maria has no reservation about offering encouragement to teen moms.

"Every child born is good news. Whether this baby was wanted or not, whether the mother is happy about her situation or not, it's *fait accompli*. A baby is on the way. We have to move forward in the most positive way possible. The last thing we want is for these babies to end up in foster care."

She would know. Maria and her husband have fostered twenty-six children over the years, even crack babies whom she cradled and soothed while they went through drug withdrawal with shaking, fevers, seizures. Even after a child leaves, Maria still holds each one in her heart. "I think about them, wonder how they're doing, who's saying I love you, who tucks them in at night. Some stay in touch with us. We attended a wedding recently."

On the way to our next stop, Maria tells me her dream is to create a home where single mothers could stay as long as they need, have a healthy pregnancy and a safe delivery. It would be run by mothers and fathers who would teach these young mothers to mother their babies. "It would set them up to succeed at the most important job in the world – being a parent."

Of course, sometimes a young, single mother decides the best thing is to let the baby go. Maria tells me about one teen who knew she wasn't ready to be a mom. She was adamant that she wouldn't leave the hospital with the baby and has never looked back.

"This choice is preferable to mothers whose babies are with them but are not thriving, or mothers who neglect their children, like the one who didn't bother to fill a prescription for asthma medication and the child went into respiratory arrest. There was one child who kept running away from home, looking for me. I always knew how the children had been treated in the homes they'd come from by watching how they played with their dolls and teddy bears. Observing them in the schoolyard during recess is also very revealing about a child."

She's wistful and fierce, determined that babies, children, and their young mothers get the nurturing they need. "We never had a lot in our house but the kids made me feel rich. Our home was always a fun place. The most important thing is connecting with others. *Relationships.*"

She says that word like she's savouring the taste of something delicious.

"My dream is to end the legacy of foster care," she says with sad determination. "Of course, there are good foster parents, but I've seen some scary things."

What she takes me to next is the opposite of scary — *safe and secure*.

It's late evening, so this will be a short visit to a single mother with three children who has a home of her own, thanks to a partnership between VON and Habitat for Humanity.

"When they contacted us, we put the word out for a family in great need. There are homeless young moms who live on the streets, in parks or shelters."

Thérèse has an infant, a ten-year-old girl, and a thirteen-year-old boy whom she had at sixteen. Her husband left after the baby was born. They were living in a rat-infested, poorly heated fire trap above a store in the worst part of town. They slept on the floor, had little food, no phone, no lock on the door. The son didn't complain, but often stayed out of the house, sometimes all night.

"This house is a hand-up, not a hand-out," Maria emphasizes. Thérèse works as a health care aide in a nursing home and pays six hundred dollars a month toward the mortgage. She also makes "sweat equity" payments by doing five hundred hours of volunteer work in the community.

"When Maria told me I'd been chosen, it was the happiest day of my life." Thérèse's face shines at her unbelievable good fortune. "I never dreamed I'd have a house. I still can't believe it's mine. 'Is this house ours?' my son kept asking, over and over, the day we moved in."

"Mommy was crying when we got the house," her daughter pipes up.

Thérèse guides me on a room-by-room tour of the small, tidy house, decorated with exuberance. "The kids chose the colours."

Ahh . . . that would explain the lemon meringue pie living room walls, her daughter's cotton candy room, and her son's Froot Loop palette. Entering each room reignites her high-wattage smile. She beams with joy; she's queen of her castle. Her happy face tells the truth of the old adage that there really is no place like home.

"Such a worthy candidate, *n'est-ce pas?*" Maria says.

After that full day of listening and travelling, I planned to sleep in, have a leisurely brunch, relax, then take a taxi to the airport for my afternoon flight home, but no – *mais non* – they won't hear of it. Rob Zwicker, nurse manager, is waiting for me in his office with coffee and croissants at eight a.m. Later, he'll give me a ride to the airport. For now, he has more to show me.

Rob reminds me of myself a few months ago when he says, "I swore I'd never work in the community. I had no interest in it. My whole career has been critical care. My hospital friends don't take my work seriously. They're dealing with ventilated patients, trauma, moose accidents. They're saving lives and –"

"Moose accidents?" I interrupt.

"Yes, especially this time of the year, there are a lot of moose-related injuries. With their non-reflective eyes and dark colour you don't see them until you suddenly plow into them. Whenever I see one, I always think, Whose life is that moose going to take?"

I have never actually seen a moose, not even in a zoo. What kind of a Canadian am I?

Rob was a manager of the emergency department at a hospital and knew nothing about maternal care, immunizations, or mental health – the specialty programs in this community – but he learned. "Even though it's not life or death like in the ICU, it's no less important. The first thing you notice outside the hospital is happy nurses. There's none of the negativity and complaining about being stressed that you hear all the time in the hospital. It's a well-kept secret that the community is a great place to work, supportive and fun."

We walk out to the parking lot to drive to our next stop. "We butter our bread differently out here," Rob says, looking proud and giving me a playful wink.

I don't know if the buttering of the bread refers to working in the community or the province of New Brunswick. Come to think of it, probably both.

In the car, Rob asks if I got to see everything I wanted to see.

"Not quite. I'd like to see a moose. Can you arrange that for me before I leave?"

"I'll see what I can do." He laughs at my little joke, but tops it with a much funnier one.

"Someone here in town called 911 to ask that a deer crossing be moved because it was interfering with traffic. 'Have them cross at a different intersection, where there's less traffic.'"

On the door of the Travel Clinic, a sign says in French and English, "Please make an appointment with the nurse." I meet a retired couple, snowbirds, planning a Caribbean cruise in a few weeks, over New Years. Luckily, it's after hurricane season, Nurse Louise says. She tells them what shots they need and the precautions they must take in various ports of call. She knows all about the titres, interactions of various meds and vaccines, stuff I know nothing about. "No one ever remembers what shots they've had," she says, "but I can sort that out." Louise echoes Rob's sentiments. "You have to have good people skills to work here. A grumpy nurse would not fit in here, but they seem to find a place for themselves in the hospital, *n'est-ce pas*?"

I remind Rob that I have to get to the airport, my flight leaves in a few hours, but he wants to squeeze in a few more visits. He drives me to the local community centre, where I sit on the floor and immediately become absorbed in the ultra-sweetness of the babies who are sitting with their mothers. Each one ventures out, takes a step or two, falls down, looks back, and finds their way home to Mom. The mothers delight in the interaction and in their babies' successes.

There's Olivier in a *petit* Montreal Canadiens jersey; Emilie in a striped Manchester United soccer jumpsuit; Josie in a furry white coat and stunning black-and-white dress with lace. The cooing, crying,

fussing, giggling, and shrieking settles down when Maria leads the
mothers in song. Is it the music or the mothers' voices that has an
immediate, almost hypnotic effect on them, faster-acting and more
potent than any narcotic I've ever given a patient?

· *"Ou est François? . . . Nous sommes très heureux. Ou est Emilie . . ."*

*"Le petit cheval qui marche, marche, marche . . . qui trot, trot, trot . . .
qui gallop . . ."*

"Papillons dans le ciel, près du sol, papillons, partout . . ."

"Songs are the best way for a baby to learn," Maria says.

I loved the baby stage with each of my sons, but looking back, I
probably spent too much time worrying if I was doing everything right,
fretting over my lost freedom and grumbling about the drudgery of
being at home, alone with a baby and then with two. I didn't appreciate
those days at the time as much as I appreciate them now, looking back
and reminiscing.

I look at my watch and remind Rob that I have to get to the airport soon.

"Don't worry, if you arrive a few minutes before your flight, that will
be enough time."

I guess it's not like the Toronto Pearson International Airport,
where you have to wait in long lines for baggage handling and to go
through the security check.

We pull into the parking lot of the local waste-management facility,
known as "The Dump." Nurse Monique Godin, an occupational health
nurse, offers biometric screening tests to identify early signs of diabetes, hypertension, and cardiac risk factors, and to screen for hepatitis
and tetanus. Based on the results, she offers individual counselling,
health teaching, and support to quit smoking. It seems to me like basic
self-care, but as Monique points out, many of the workers here are
uneducated, even illiterate. Many are willing to do work most Canadians
won't touch. Some are First Nations people, others are undocumented
workers with no Canadian health insurance, refugees from war-torn
countries, or simply unaware of health practices most of us consider
"basic," like a nutritious diet, hand washing, and hygiene.

"They don't understand the risks of toxic substances," she says.

The risks she's referring to become immediately clear when Monique takes me to the trash sorting area. Some of the items that have shown up in the trash that workers handle and sort: a skinned dog, deer heads (there's a taxidermist in town), sea flares, mouldy furniture, the remains of a grenade, explosives, unidentified chemicals, used syringes and needles, and contaminated toys.

"Even though they're dealing with such yucky stuff, it's still hard to impress upon them the importance of wearing gloves and a mask. They don't get it, so they don't bother."

Some of their basic needs have never been addressed.

"Most have never seen a doctor or nurse before. Never had a checkup or immunizations. Many need dental work, glasses, or hearing aids. You can see how you can make a huge impact on their lives, and their ability to get educated, by getting these primary health needs met."

Monique is also a home care nurse who visits veterans, young and old, active and retired from duty; many suffer post-traumatic stress disorder from wars, both current and past. They have chronic pain, fragile mental health, and substance abuse problems. One client is a forty-one-year-old veteran who served in Afghanistan. His wife left him shortly after he returned home – damaged and shell-shocked, angry and depressed. He suffers from nightmares and wakes up screaming, feeling like he's being choked.

"He has flashbacks to crowds of women begging for food, then later seeing them murdered. He has a recurrent nightmare of children being murdered, others horrifically injured – one who had a bomb blow up in her face. Now he has a cocaine addiction and recently took an overdose in a suicide attempt. He gets agitated, but I never feel threatened in his presence. We've built a trust, he and I, you see."

The mental health issues that Monique identified in her practice gave rise to an initiative that Rob tells me about on the way to the airport. Directed by Karen Ursel, a nursing professor at the University of

Moncton, they've created a support group where people with depression can share their experiences; no doctor's diagnosis or referral is
required. Depression was chosen as the focus because, according to
the World Health Organization, it's the leading mental health problem
in the world, and the number-one cause of disability to work.

"For our purposes, depression is whatever the person says they
feel. We ask simple questions like, 'What does living with depression
mean to you?' or 'How does depression impact your life?'" Rob hands
me a sheaf of papers that compile the responses.

"No energy. I want to sleep all day."

"It makes me feel like I'm a zombie, or the walking dead."

"I want to be left alone, yet feel rejected when left alone."

"I can't do my job because the smallest things seem insurmountable."

"I want to sleep all day, not wake up. I feel disconnected from
everything and everyone."

"I've lived all my life with depression and have tried so hard to hide it."

Depression can lead to absenteeism or "presentism," Rob says,
"where people show up in the workplace, but are not engaged or not
working to full capacity or potential. All you have to do is listen to a
mentally ill person describe what they feel and share their story and
you get it. This is not about trying harder or behaving better. It's an
illness that needs treatment."

"What treatment do you offer?"

"Connection is the main one. Listening, another. On a practical
level, we make referrals to doctors, talk a lot about self-care, like exercise and diet, and also explore the meaning of their depression with
them. We constantly ask, 'What would be most helpful to you?' One
thing that emerged from asking that question was the consensus that
they wanted a support group. We set one up. We advertised it and waited,
but no one came."

"Too depressed?" (This is a joke that only someone who's experienced depression can get away with.)

"The stigma kept them away. But we knew there was a problem

because the nurses were identifying it. In some cases, a home care nurse was their only connection. But we want every door a person goes to to seek help to be the right door."

Rob gets me to the airport a few minutes before my flight, which is plenty of time to zip through security and board the plan. Settled in my seat beside the window, I munch on a sandwich Maria made for me. I can't wait to get home and see my family after being away for two weeks. Maybe I'll fit in a few ICU shifts, just so they don't forget me.

The plane gains momentum and lifts up to the sky. I look down at the patchwork of fields and farmhouses, isolated and remote from each other, and the wide expanses of forest and wild bush in between and all around. The ground below recedes and the houses and trees become smaller. Suddenly, I look down and see – I spot the antlers first, lumbering through trees – it's the size of a plastic toy animal. Yes, I'm sure – it's a moose! My moose.

15

BACK AT THE RANCH

HOME SWEET HOME. It's great to be back with my husband and kids. They're happy and flourishing and didn't seem to miss me too much (was my absence even noticed?), so no worries there. I've been away for only a few weeks, but after going so many places, meeting so many people, and hearing so many stories, it feels much longer. The stories have changed me. I'm not the same person, or the same nurse. But there's no time to reflect on that because a day after I arrive, I receive news that's first shocking, then disappointing.

First, the shocking part. Judith called. I went into my office and closed the door so there'd be no noise or distractions. I need to have my wits about me when I speak to Judith. Just as I'm about to ask where she is – Moscow? Rio de Janeiro? – she gets to the reason for her call.

"I've resigned as chief of VON. I'm leaving the organization."

"What will happen to VON?" *What's happening with my trip?*

"There are many capable people in this organization, as you know. I will stay on in an emeritus role and VON will manage just fine without me."

"Why are you leaving?"

"I want to focus on my campaign for president of the International Council of Nurses."

Yes, it makes sense. She once told me she never stays in any position more than a few years, sufficient time for her to make her unique contribution. Then it's time to move on to the next challenge. But what about the fate of my epic odyssey? I'm still looking forward to getting out west to British Columbia, to Alberta, to Newfoundland and, of course, Thunder Bay. But next comes the disappointing news. VON is in crisis. This venerable institution has fallen on hard times financially. Cutbacks in programs and staff layoffs are in the works. Until further notice, there is a freeze on unnecessary expenses and a travel ban. As for me, my trip is to be drastically curtailed to the few local, remaining visits that have already been arranged. The last leg of my journey will be a stripped-down roadshow with only a few more stops.

That's it? No Rockies or Prairies? No Thunder Bay? And, of course, New York was taken.

"Go with the flow," my husband says, and, of course, he's right.

A pile of letters from Audrey accumulated while I was away. She's stepped it up. They used to arrive about once a month, then once a week, but six have arrived in the past two weeks while I've been gone. I wrote her one letter before I left for Nova Scotia, but long ago gave up trying to respond to each one. Who can keep up with Audrey? Even my kids recognize the familiar, primly embellished script with its precise return to the line, as if a ruler were placed underneath, and, of course, the daisies, cupcakes, clowns, sea horses, balloons, and dragons.

I settle in with a cup of tea on the couch to read.

Thank you for your exhilarating, but undated note. . . . Why haven't you provided answers to my most pressing questions?
1. Did you work on both Christmas and New Year's Day?
2. When will you send me a picture of you in the sweater Nurse Stephanie knitted for you?

———

. . . I received a special gift for Christmas – pneumonia. My blood sugar soared tragically and Hilda suspected I was harbouring an infection. They ambulanced me off to the hospital. I was very happy and peaceful knowing that I was finally going, this time for good. How does one cope gracefully with the oxygen mask while still keeping up conversation and eating chocolate for energy? An antibiotic was prescribed and bed rest, too, but what I need is eternal rest. They used to call pneumonia the "old person's friend." But my earthly friends took on the Pneumonia Project and rescued me. I'm back home now but in a devastatingly debilitated state.

My back is wickedly weak and the left leg attached to it is slowing down. But I'm a good patient and don't need much care at all, just water and feeding like a hardy house plant.

. . . Yes, they recycled me, gave me a new transmission and now I'm back in the garage – I mean at home. I'm still alive at everyone's request. At least, I am trying to do my best.

My caregivers have installed a raised toilet seat to assist me in those matters. It is cumbersome. I miss my old one. Perhaps you'll come and give me a demo how to work it?

It is January 6th, exactly one month to my party. I will try to hang on, but because it is wise, I plan for my demise. (After the party.) I expect you to be there. Don't let me down.

I get stationery, a pen, a stamp, and an envelope to write back. *Question: Who will inherit your sticker collection?*

Back at the ranch.

I never realized the extent to which the hospital is not a cheery place. As I walked in this morning at the start of a twelve-hour day shift, I noticed, as if seeing for the first time, that there are a lot of tense, grim people around here, and I'm not talking about the patients. As for me,

I'm back in the groove, in my element. Ahh, the symphony of beeps, buzzes, the ringing of alarms, the overhead staticky announcements, the rushing high-heeled footsteps, phones ringing at the nursing station, the nerve-jangling hustle and bustle – it's music to my ears. I'd been hoping for an exciting day and it looks promising. Someone is crashing (the arrest cart has just been wheeled in), there's someone down in the ER who needs an ICU bed but we're full so he'll have to be "bed-spaced" to the cardiovascular ICU for now. Three patients are on ECLS, each requiring two nurses assigned to their care. There's a young woman admitted overnight with viral myocarditis who's in florid septic shock and respiratory failure. Another patient is in hepatic failure and is deeply unresponsive from an encephalopathic coma. His family sits by his bed, guiltily hoping for an inevitable tragedy that might bring a liver transplant to save their son's life. An eighty-three-year-old man was in the ER for six hours overnight until he was stable enough to be moved to the ICU. He has lung cancer and massive pleural effusions and abscesses on his lungs. "Please try to save his life," the family implored. The team did that, but unfortunately he died in the elevator on the way to the ICU. (This was awful for the family, but it does mean that at least there will be a spot for the bed-spaced patient in CV ICU.)

"Technically, we just admitted a dead man," was the night nurse's rueful comment.

A fifty-year-old man has a respiratory infection and thanks to the tragic lessons learned from SARS the patient's nurse and doctor didn't miss a beat. They closed the doors, put on the special, fitted masks, gowns, gloves, and eye shields, turned on the reverse air filter system, and taped "Airborne Isolation" signs outside his room.

In short – an ordinary ICU day.

At lunch, I catch up on the news. A week ago Richard Thornton-Sharp was admitted to the ICU in respiratory failure. He's back home, but now needs around-the-clock care. His husband, Jim, called the ICU to tell us that Richard stays in bed now, too weak to even sit up. Jim has taken a leave of absence from his job to take care of Richard full-time. With home care assistance, Richard is now receiving palliative care.

I wonder if I'll see him again.

Later in the afternoon, when the daily, predictable hypoglycemic slump hits and our stress levels peak, each of us finds a moment to dart into our manager Denise's office (where the door is always open) and dip into the glass bowl of chocolates she keeps on her desk. Here's an interesting research question: Is there a correlation between our stress levels and the chocolate level in the jar? I hypothesize an indirect correlation; as one goes up, the other goes down. Mmmmmm. Perhaps I can get a government grant – or a chocolate manufacturer – to subsidize this worthwhile investigation.

It's great to be back, but as my shift comes to an end, for the first time I wonder if "excitement" might be overrated. Is "excitement" the essential ingredient for a meaningful career, for work that matters? Is constant action, high-stakes drama, adrenaline rushes, et al. – and the stress we complain about, but, I suspect, actually relish, even crave – what it takes to make a job satisfying?

Now the ICU seems a smaller, more contained world than my new, expansive one. I'm looking forward to getting back on the road, to the world beyond the hospital. Just as I love my hospital world, I've grown to love this other world. I'm discovering that helping people live their lives can be as *exciting* as saving those lives – not to mention all the *fun* of being on the road as a roving nurse-reporter. In fact, I'm leaving tomorrow for Ottawa, to see what VON has to show me there. Just when I think I've seen all there is, they surprise me with something new.

16

THE FAR, DARK SIDE

STATISTICS USUALLY MAKE my eyes glaze over and my mind go blank, but these ones make me sit up and take notice, perhaps because I can now visualize what they actually look like.

"The unpaid labour of family caregivers saves our health care system twenty-five billion dollars a year." "Over three million Canadians provide informal caregiving to a family member. . . . Twelve per cent of children or teenagers provide significant care to family members."

Child caregivers? Say it isn't so.

Full disclosure: I was a child caregiver to my mother, but I didn't always carry out my role with a skip in my step and a song in my heart. So, I guess I have an interest in the topic.

In the Ottawa office of Bonnie Schroeder, director of caregiving for VON Canada, a poster says, "Are you a caregiver? You are if you think you are." Another reads, "Are you a caregiver? Chances are you are. Or will be. At some point, we are all called upon to be caregivers." That's true, but not everyone is up for the challenge. What I do know is that everyone has somebody they're worried about.

I know some incredible family caregivers. My close friend Jasna cares for her profoundly developmentally delayed twenty-year-old son at home on her days off from work. Together with her husband, Jack, and their other two children, they dress and feed Alex, and medicate him when he has one of many daily seizures.

"You do what you gotta do," Jasna always says, brushing off my expressions of admiration for the way her family deals with their situation.

You do what you gotta do.

I suppose that's true, but not everyone does it as wholeheartedly or as graciously as the caregivers I've met on this journey. Sure, they have their bad days, but mostly they hunker down – with few complaints, endless patience, and little self-pity. Their nobility appears to be effortless. I admire these caregivers but I understand and identify more with those who struggle with the role. For me, it's not difficult to imagine how a well-meaning caregiver could become a frustrated, resentful, neglectful – or even abusive – caregiver. As for someone forced into the role? I have great sympathy; it's hard enough to be a good caregiver when you take on the role willingly. I'm hoping that Bonnie will speak candidly about this dark side of caregiving – not just the blessings, but its burdens, too.

She doesn't disappoint.

"'Overwhelmed' is the word you constantly hear," Bonnie says. She gives me a folder full of research articles about the higher incidence of impaired immune systems, depression, infectious diseases, and premature aging. One study from the Faculty of Nursing at the University of Western Ontario found that 40 per cent of nurses are double-duty caregivers. This is the highest percentage across all professions. These nurses are fulfilling both professional and family caregiving roles simultaneously, around the clock, shift after shift, without a break.

"Caregivers feel invisible. They are rarely asked how they are doing. The focus is always on the patient. I always say if they've taken their pills, are clean, dressed, and made it to an appointment, it's because of caregivers. But many are pushed to the brink and end up compromising their own health and jeopardizing their jobs, too."

Many people are not prepared for the hands-on work of caregiving. Bonnie tells about a man who cared for his wife after a stroke. When a home care worker visited, she noticed bruises on her neck and brought it to the husband's attention. "She had a poo," the husband said in explanation. "What's wrong with that?" she asked. "On the carpet," he said, looking remorseful. The home care worker reported the incident, which led to providing respite and support for the husband. Maybe those measures ultimately saved the woman's life.

Pee and poo are a big deal; for many, they are a game changer. "I'd kept them at home until that," I've heard caregivers say. Incontinence draws a line in the sand. "When it happens, you're never ready," the son of an ICU patient once told me. "I can cope with anything but that."

We're unused to tending the human body, yet we accept handling our dog's excrement and have little trouble with babies' diapers. What happens to make us become repulsed, squeamish, even claim a constitutional inability to handle the body's messes? Love can only get you so far.

According to Bonnie, "respite" is their number-one need. A husband who came to Bonnie in despair said he found himself getting aggressive toward his wife, who had Alzheimer's. When she started going to an adult day program, he finally got a break. He's taken up golf again, having lunch with friends. "It gave me back my life," he said. The benefits to the wife were significant, too. "I've seen it with my own eyes: ADPs save lives," Bonnie says.

It's what we say about hospital care, but now I realize that both claims are correct.

Bonnie invites me for lunch, but I excuse myself. I have other plans. I want to take a walk, stroll around downtown Ottawa. See the Rideau Canal, the Parliament Buildings, but first, I have a stop to make. It's only a few blocks from the VON office to Elgin Street where Perfect Books is located. Hopefully, the owner, Jim Sherman, will be there.

The sign over the door says, "A Proudly Canadian . . . Fiercely Independent Bookstore." It's one of the few small, independent bookstores left in the world. They're a dying breed – as are fanatic readers like Jim and me. Inside the shop, classical music is playing softly and the patrons are whispering as if the place is holy, except what's worshipped here are the words, ideas, and stories contained in these pages. Jim stocks the latest bestsellers alongside hand-picked, lesser-known titles from up-and-coming writers, on smooth pine shelves. Best of all, Jim is here to talk books. He's been my bookseller at conferences where I was the speaker, and in his store, he always keeps copies of *A Nurse's Story* in stock.

We stand at the front display window where sunlight pours in, warming the store on this frigid day, and we launch right into discussing our mixed feelings about the new Jonathan Franzen, to going into raptures over Alice Munro, as always, and to anticipating the soon-to-be-released Vincent Lam. We compare "To Read" lists, lament classics we still haven't gotten around to, and share book jokes, like the one about the customer who came into the store recently and innocently asked Jim, "Do you have any books by Jane Eyre?"

Something outside in front of the store catches Jim's eye because he stops talking mid-book to peer out the window. He shields his eyes from the bright sun and looks perturbed. I look out, too, to see what he sees. But there's nothing there except for a pile of garbage bags, old rags, and cardboard boxes strewn about on the sidewalk. I hadn't noticed it there when I walked into the store a few minutes ago, but it's hard to miss now.

Jim raps on the window. Suddenly, the heap of trash moves. I look closer. Horrified, I see that there's a human being under there. He sits up and looks drowsy, like he's been awakened. He holds on to an empty beer bottle. A bedraggled, grimy person has set up base camp and taken shelter under the awning of Perfect Books. Clearly concerned, Jim calls a nearby shelter to have someone come and escort him away.

"Not a customer, I presume?" I quip.

"No, but he is a regular. He likes this spot outside my door because there's a sewer grate right there that he lies on for the warmth on a cold day like this."

I wonder why he can't just stay there, if it's warm and protected. Where is he supposed to go if he doesn't have a home? But I also see it from Jim's point of view. This person's shocking appearance might deter customers from entering the shop, and we all know bookstores need all the customers they can get to survive.

"Bad for business, I guess?" I say.

"Yes, but lying there isn't good for him, either. It's no way for a human being to live. It's freezing out there and he needs a meal and a place to stay tonight."

Probably not just tonight. Likely tomorrow night, too.

So many times I've looked away and walked on by. It's getting harder to do that now.

Later in the afternoon, I return to the office ready to meet a VON client that Bonnie has invited to talk with me. Georgina McPhee cared for her husband, who died last year. She's fifty now, but when she and her husband were in their mid-forties, he developed early-onset dementia, and his decline was fast and drastic.

Georgina is a slight sad-looking woman, attractive with no makeup or jewellery, in a ballerina chignon, loose tendrils at the sides of her face, wearing a long velvet skirt and a romantic shawl around her shoulders. She is ready to share her experience and does so with unflinching honesty.

"It started off as mild confusion, but soon Allan couldn't follow TV or keep up a conversation. Here he was, a brilliant university professor in the prime of his life, and almost overnight, he became a helpless, needy child. He had always been meticulous about his appearance, but soon became slovenly, not brushing his teeth or showering. He kept asking questions over and over. 'Why is there a light in the doorbell? Why is there a light in the car? Make it stop. Make it stop.'"

"Did you ever get a break?"

"Only when I put on repetitive children's TV shows or a movie with a familiar plot. It soothed him momentarily, but then he'd panic and call out for me, not realizing I was in the next room or the kitchen. He kept launching into long stories. The children took the photos off the piano because that would get him started. He teased them inappropriately. He could no longer play the card games we loved. When we went out he'd make rude comments about someone's appearance and people looked at me like, 'Can't you control him?,' so we stopped socializing to avoid embarrassment. Our world shrank. I became housebound, a prisoner in my own home.

"Then he started using the wastebasket in our bedroom as a toilet. Each time he did that I'd want to scream. I'd have to go into another room to collect myself but he'd follow me there."

Georgina shifts in her chair, but I don't move a muscle. I'm mainlining her story, totally riveted by her courage in telling it so honestly.

"*It's not him, it's the disease*, I kept telling myself. Here was his warm body right beside me, but he was gone. It wasn't him. Sex? Forget that. He was my child. He couldn't be a father. The kids referred to him as 'this dad' or the 'real dad,' or the 'new dad' or the 'old dad.' I was a single mom, on my own . . ."

For Georgina, one of the hardest things was her husband's "importuning." I didn't think I knew the meaning of that word, but when she describes the behaviour, I realize I do.

"He looked to me for constant attention. He wanted me to entertain him. He needed endless reassurance and encouragement. He'd call out for me, ask me questions, and follow me around. He would stand outside the bathroom, asking, 'When are you coming out? When are you coming out?' So many times I felt I couldn't take it anymore, but I did, for six long years.

"One advantage of my situation was that I never had to wonder what to do each day."

(That's a joke you can make only if you've been a caregiver yourself.)

Georgina learned to take help whenever it was offered, even from strangers, until her husband became wary of unfamiliar people in the house.

"'Who's here? They're stealing the TV,' he'd say over and over. He was even suspicious of his own reflection in the mirror. He thought someone was spying on him.

"I felt so alone, until one day, my sister, who is a nurse, came for a visit. After two days watching me she said, 'I don't know how you've managed this far.'"

"I'm also a nurse who's wondering the same thing," I say.

"'It's time, Georgina,' my sister said. 'He's too much for you. You need to put him in a nursing home.' What a relief to hear her say it. It's only when others get a glimpse into your world that they finally get what you're going through. I had enormous guilt over that decision and tortured myself with questions. Could I have been a better caregiver? Did I do enough? Could I have kept him at home longer? I kept thinking, *I should be able to manage this myself*.

"The standard is higher for family than professionals. The expectation is that because you love him, you can cope with anything – annoying behaviours, aggressiveness, incontinence, bowel movements. I would look at him and all I could see was someone I had to take care of. I was his babysitter. No one saw that my marriage was over. His body was there, but I was alone. He was gone. I began to resent – even hate – him. I couldn't feel the love I once had for him. Without his income or mine anymore, the financial stress was enormous. One thing that helped was the day program for him and a spousal support group for me. I had errands to do but I needed the support group more. We talked about everything and everyone understood because they were going through the same thing. We could complain about no more sex or confess our murderous thoughts about having to clean them up or that we wished it were over. It's not that we wanted the person to die, only for the suffering to end."

Now Georgina comes to a part of her story that is difficult to tell. She tenses up and pulls back. Hesitating. I can see her thinking whether to divulge this part or not. She looks at me for a moment, trying to judge if it is safe for her to say it. She goes for it.

"There was one day I'll never forget. Allan was calling out for me and following me around the house, and suddenly, I lost control of myself. I grabbed his shoulders, slammed him up against a wall, and yelled, 'Listen to me! Would you stop this? I can't take it anymore.' We had always been gentle and loving toward each other. I was appalled at what I was capable of. It was abuse, plain and simple, but we all have our limits. We have to be able to say, 'I need help.'"

Georgina wants to support other family caregivers, so when I ask her what helps, she is ready with her response.

"First of all, make sure you *see* the caregiver, not just the patient. Remember to ask, 'How are *you* doing?' and then sit and listen. Don't ever say, 'What can I do to help?' It's vague and the person is too overwhelmed to think of something. They'll always say, 'No thanks,' or 'I'm fine,' but don't believe them. Nothing could be further from the truth. They are using every bit of their energy to simply keep it together. They can't come up with something to suggest. Instead, say 'I'll look after this,' or 'I'll do this.' Just tell me what you're going to do and do it. Or, show up and figure out what's needed. Weed the garden, walk the dog, bring a meal. Do what needs doing."

There's more.

"Being careful with words is important. Your words can heal or harm. People say such thoughtless things. You're an open wound, so you take everything to heart. When I finally took my husband to a nursing home, there was a father with a son who had multiple sclerosis. The nurse said to me, 'You have no idea how hard it is for him,' totally discounting my situation and how hard it was for me. You never know what another person is facing."

She advises caregivers to find hope in realistic, achievable goals, because they always feel they're not doing enough and should be doing more. "Tell them they are doing enough. Sometimes all I could manage was to keep Allan safe and clean. Remind caregivers that they have rights – the right not to get burnt out, to take care of themselves, to not be left financially destitute. I'll never forget the family who spent thousands of dollars to retrofit their home and put in wheelchair ramps, safety bars, and an electronic lift. They brought their father home and he died a day later. Families have the right not to become bankrupt. They have a right to breaks from caregiving to rest and renew themselves. Many caregivers do too much, to the detriment of their health. Caregivers need to learn practical strategies for coping."

On a larger scale, there's a need for more day programs, especially for children and young adults with autism spectrum disorder or developmental delays, and group homes for young adults with developmental disabilities or mental illness. Georgina feels strongly that these places must be aesthetically pleasing, not old or depressing, and filled with art, music, and beautiful things. The people who work there must have a sense of purpose and pride.

"We need to check in with caregivers and be aware of their capacities and needs. Sometimes, it's not the patient who is suffering the most."

You do what you gotta do. It's a phrase that echoes in my mind after I say goodbye to Georgina and walk back to my hotel. Yes, it's true. However, you have a choice *how* you do it, and in my experience, the best caregivers do it with loving kindness to themselves first, so that they then are able to offer the same to the ones in their care.

When Bonnie had told me about the high incidence of young caregivers, I wondered about the effect upon children and teenagers of having such heavy and mature responsibilities. "How does it affect them in the long run?" I ask her. "Does it make them become more compassionate human beings or traumatize them for life?"

"It's not the age of the caregiver, or the form that the caregiving takes," she said. "It is what the individual experiences and how it affects that person."

To speak directly with child caregivers, Bonnie suggests I call Denise Clayton, the mother in a family whose child, Stephanie, was born with an omphalocele, a condition where her intestines were located outside her body. Now she's twelve, and, after many surgeries, Stephanie continues to have numerous medical problems and nutritional issues. When Denise and I first talk on the phone, I'm surprised to hear her mention the benefits of their situation first. "It's made our family stronger. It's given the children confidence and a sense of accomplishment." She says she'd like to meet with me but apologizes that she can't. Between caring for Stephanie, informing her teachers about her illness, making frequent runs to the hospital, and trying to keep life somewhat normal for Sydney, aged fourteen, and Danielle, aged ten, she has no spare time. Denise suggests I email my questions to her daughters. "They'll be thrilled you want to hear from them. It's usually Stephanie who gets all the attention."

So, I start up a correspondence with Sydney and Danielle Clayton, who are very pleased to respond to my inquiries.

WHAT'S IT LIKE BEING A CAREGIVER TO YOUR SISTER?

SYDNEY: Good evening. My name is Sydney Anna Clayton. As you may have heard, I am Stephanie's older sister. What's it like being her caregiver? Stressful! But no matter how tiring, difficult, or frustrating it may be at times – well, most of the time – there's not a better feeling in the world to finally see her smiling face when she gets a moment of relief from her suffering.

DANIELLE: Hi, I'm Danielle. You never know if she is going to be happy or mad or sensitive or grumpy. Maybe start out normal then five minutes later she freaks out and you can't go near her.

WHAT ARE SOME OF THE THINGS YOU DO TO HELP CARE FOR YOUR SISTER?

SYDNEY: In my experience, the best way to help is to stay away, but be around when she needs cheering up. As the oldest, I have always been the one to protect her, clown around with her, cheer her up, inspire her, be a role model, teach her how to be a regular kid. I helped her work on her "swag factor" and be the person I knew she was. Fortunately, I never had to take care of her medically, but knowing how difficult it is just being her support system, I can't

imagine how stressful it would be to take care of her medical
needs as well.

DANIELLE: If she's tired I watch Movies with her if she wants to play I
play with her if she got admitted to hospital I will beg to visit her
and if she is also admitted to hospital I bring her clothes and toys
called American girls I bring her some.

ARE THERE ANY GOOD OR FUN PARTS ABOUT HAVING A SISTER WHO NEEDS YOUR HELP?

SYDNEY: I would like to make it clear that having a relative that's so
critically ill, is no situation I would wish upon passing over to
another person. It is not fun or enjoyable. However, if I were to say
that it has never changed my personal life or my family for the
better, I would be lying. It's forced me to grow up fast. At age two,
instead of thinking what kind of cookie I wanted for dessert, I was
learning how to pronounce "omphalocele." You can imagine how
difficult it was trying to understand this complicated word when I
was still trying to figure out why the swings moved the way they did.
Being an older sister to a sick child has made me more patient,
calm, courageous, and less selfish. So there are positive aspects.

DANIELLE: Well some fun things are that we are not ever bored cause
you have a job to do. You have more fun cause your always busy and
you have many more opportunities.

WHAT ARE THE HARD PARTS?

SYDNEY: It's always difficult. There is never a break. Stephanie has pain
that NEVER goes away and must always be dealt with. Steph has been
through a lot and it is difficult to keep her cool at times. You can see
in her eyes how hard it is for her. Having a sister like Steph has never
been easy. It's not easy for even the smartest of doctors to understand
her. There is nothing we can do and nowhere that we can go that is
not affected by Stephanie's health. There is no minute of this life that
I do not think about Steph. It is difficult not knowing what the future

holds. With Steph it is not possible to go day by day. It's more of an hourly thing. Everything has to be planned by the second and organized so tediously to avoid mess-ups or accidents or danger.

DANIELLE: Well, one of my fears are when she is really sick in the hospital or when she has been naughty and got grounded she gets mad easily and scares everyone in the house.

ARE THERE TIMES WHEN YOU DON'T WANT TO BE A CAREGIVER?

SYDNEY: I feel this often. There are times I wish I could be a kid with no responsibilities, no worries, live a carefree life. I try to cherish the good times and make them last because you never know when it could all come to an end.

DANIELLE: Well, sometimes. Let's say you're playing a game and she has to be a certain colour, so I give in because she's sick. If she gets mad, I get scared something will happen.

It's not about what they do, but about how they are affected.

17

THE WAY A HUG MATTERS

JUST BEFORE I LEFT OTTAWA, Bonnie told me about another appointment she'd set up for me. I'd had enough by then and just wanted to get home, but she was insistent.

"There are some situations that are beyond what family caregiving can do. Even those who want to do it all simply can't, and they require professional nursing in the home."

She handed me a piece of paper with an address of a client I was to meet at his home, early the next morning. I was tired and just wanted to be on my way. I considered cancelling, but it was conveniently located along my drive back to Toronto and since Bonnie had gone to the trouble to it set up, I felt guilty not going through with it.

It's only now, three weeks later, that I am able to put into words what I experienced there.

———

I pulled into a long driveway where two pink tricycles were parked alongside an SUV. Bonnie told me only that I'd be meeting the client Gaétan Tremblay, that his wife was a high-powered corporate lawyer named Veronique, and that he had identical twin five-year-old girls. A stunning woman in a leather bomber jacket and tall leather boots, carrying a bulging briefcase, emerged from the house, and I assumed she was Veronique. In the midst of talking on the phone, she stopped to call out to me. "Hi! You must be the nurse here to see Gaétan. Go on in. The door is open. He's expecting you." She waved to me as she backed out on to the street. I pulled into her spot.

It was 7:30 in the morning, but Nurse Rhonda Jacquard was already there and busy with Gaétan's nursing care in the bedroom. She came out to introduce herself and tell me a little bit about her client. A year and a half ago, Gaétan was in a freak accident that left him paralyzed from the neck down. He's now a quadriplegic and requires six hours of nursing care a day – three in the morning and three in the evening – 365 days a year; not a day can be missed.

Gaétan was still in bed, she said, and she'd call out to me to come in after a few minutes more, when they'd finished his morning care and bowel routine.

He must have autonomic dysfunction, I thought – most quads and some paras do. When the central nervous system doesn't function properly, the muscles are affected, including those of the gastrointestinal tract. They slow down and don't move as effectively. The person cannot evacuate stool and so, every day, it must be eased out with an enema or extracted manually.

Rhonda called me to come in. The bedroom was dim; the shades were drawn. Gaétan lay flat on his back and lifted his head to greet me and say, "hey" when I walked in. I introduced myself and he invited me to sit down, but I didn't know where, as Rhonda was using the only chair in the room to place her supplies upon. Gaétan turned his head and nodded over at the opposite side of the bed, his wife's side. I wanted to respect his personal space, but there was nowhere else to sit and I didn't want to talk to him standing up, looking down at him lying down, so I perched on the edge of the king-sized bed in Veronique's space, still warm from her recently slumbering body.

Deftly, Rhonda turned Gaétan on his side to face me so that he and I could talk face-to-face. That position also gave her better access to attend to the pressure sore on his backside. That way, she could get a good look at it, clean it, and change the dressing.

Rhonda put a pillow behind Gaétan's upper back for support and placed his arms down along his sides, and his hands and fingers in their natural positions. On his left pinky finger there was a plain, unpolished metal ring, the sign of a Canadian engineer. Upon graduation, they are allowed to wear this ring, which they receive in a secret ceremony. It's made from iron extracted from a bridge that collapsed due to a fatal engineering flaw. It's a reminder of human fallibility and the responsibility for people's lives that engineers bear.

Gaétan said that he was agreeable to this interview, but on the condition that VON will benefit from book sales. Once I had assured him that was indeed the case, we were ready to begin.

Opening my notebook and clicking my pen like an on-the-scene news reporter, moving in for the big scoop, I blurted out, "So, what happened?" Imperceptibly, he flinched. Perhaps my inexplicable nervousness was what made me so overeager. *Not a good start.* In an attempt to smother that tactless question, I rushed to cover it with an even more insensitive one. "Was it a diving accident?" Gaétan turned his head away from me. He looked up at the ceiling. It seemed like the interview was over.

"Okay. Call it a 'diving accident,'" he said, his teeth clenched.

Diving accident. I get it. The term implies recklessness. It begs the question of how an educated, intelligent person could be so careless – no, stupid – as to dive into shallow water.

I apologize. Something eases between us. He smiles at me, all is forgiven. He has a gorgeous smile and is an incredibly attractive man. Now I can see the hot, studly guy I saw in a framed photograph I was admiring on the coffee table in the living room as I was snooping around, waiting to come in to his room. In the picture, he had a guitar in one arm and the other was slung around the graceful shoulders of the gorgeous Veronique, the couple looking so happy and in love.

"My accident happened a year and a half ago. It was a warm summer evening. I'd been playing music, chillin' with friends, had a couple of drinks. I went to take a dip in the pool, but slipped off the ladder and fell on my head. In an instant, I was paralyzed. I lay there at the bottom, waiting for someone to save me. They did. Later, I wished they hadn't."

Gaétan's injury was high up on his cervical spinal cord. One vertebra higher and he'd be on a ventilator permanently, completely unable to breathe for himself, like he can now.

"Before my accident, I'd been into running and working out. I was in the best shape of my life. Now look at me." He looks down at his pale, soft body. There is no muscle tone in his legs, arms, or chest, and considerable atrophy. What a drastic change from the rugged face, the chiselled image of "before."

"I was so buff. Bodybuilding was my obsession. I played hockey, rode a motorcycle. I played guitar in a rock band. Now I can only play the harmonica."

"What was it like at first? Do you remember the hospital?"

"The ICU? It was great. Getting off of the ventilator was a wonderful feeling. My first food was a slice of watermelon and nothing ever tasted so delicious. I was confident I'd make a full recovery. I told myself that I was going to be the one to beat the odds. My mind was strong and I was in great shape, with huge muscle mass and peak cardiovascular stamina. To be completely paralyzed? It was unthinkable, totally unacceptable to me."

"What was rehab like?"

"I was very motivated and worked hard. It was a hopeful time – mostly. There was one guy there who kept trying to encourage me. 'I get the nurses to toss me Timbits,' he'd say. 'Yesterday I got three out of six in my mouth.' 'Dude, that's supposed to cheer me up?' 'Don't worry,' he said. 'I used to buy a dozen and get three in my mouth. Now, I'm three out of six.' He freaked me right out. *Keep this guy away from me. Don't let him near me again.*"

We laughed but, of course, it wasn't funny. Here's another perk of being a nurse: you can share jokes that only you and your patient get.

"In those early days, each step of the way, you can only handle a certain amount of information. There was a girl in rehab, Desdemona. Her husband left, ran off with her nurse. She was so depressed. She wouldn't exercise, didn't even try to use her arms. She retreated and was jealous of me because I could breathe. Another guy was jealous of her because she had arms, but Desi was jealous of him because he had legs and a wife. We were all jealous of the paraplegics. *They have it made. They can move their arms.* But if I was a paraplegic I'm sure I'd be unhappy, wanting to walk.

"That was rehab. Back then, I had a positive attitude. Now, I'm more scared. Suicide has been on my mind a lot lately." He looks back over his shoulder, up at Rhonda. Their eyes contain his secrets.

Has he ever asked her to help him? What would she say? What would I say if I were his nurse? "Do you have a plan how you would do it?"

"How could I do it by myself? That's the problem. Think about it. Suicide is hard for a quad. Paraplegics have more options. I came very close one day, a few months ago. I was at the girls' swimming lesson. They had gotten out of the pool and were in the change room. No one was around. I wheeled over to the deep end and stared down into the water. All I'd have to do was press the button on my chair and roll myself in. I was so close. Then I heard their voices – Juliette and Genevieve. They were giggling. They sounded so carefree. I thought about what it would do to them. To Veronique, too, but in many ways it would also make life easier for her. The girls were the main reason I didn't do it. At that point, they were the only reason. I haven't told this to anyone, other than Rhonda, of course."

What a privilege to be let in, too.

"Now my focus is getting on with life. It's a choice – get busy living or get busy dying. My chance of walking is nil. My hope is for some mobility in my arms. That would give me more independence. Meanwhile, I have lots of gadgets that help me. A pincer with a fork

attached so I can feed myself. A motorized wheelchair. A voice-acti-
vated computer. A coughing machine because I'm super-vulnerable to
infections. With winter coming, a simple cold could kill me. My cough
is weak and I can't clear my airway."

Rhonda showed me how his nurses use the device to stimulate him
to cough and expand his lungs. They do this every day, and more frequently if he has a cold.

"Recently, I developed an electrical disturbance in my heart so I
have a pacemaker. It's going to take awhile to accept my new reality. I
haven't come to terms with it yet."

I can hardly come to terms with it myself, just hearing about it.

"I've had a lot of time to think about all of this, so in a way, it's
harder now than at the beginning when I couldn't take it all in. At least
I no longer have a fear of death. I've lost that."

Rhonda has taken down the dressing and is examining the wound
on his backside. She motioned for me to take a look and Gaétan nodded
his agreement. I leaned over his hip to see an open and inflamed ulcer,
not overly large or deep, with no sign of infected discharge.

"It's getting smaller and beginning to show some granulation
tissue," Rhonda reports.

Both signs of healing.

(Hopefully, they both knew that a pressure sore like his is a practically unavoidable result of sitting in a wheelchair for most of the
hours of the day. Even Superman Christopher Reeve, who became a
quadriplegic after a horseback riding accident, and had the most
advanced equipment and the best around-the-clock nursing care,
developed pressure sores. Most people assume they're caused by bad
nursing care. Without frequent turning, proper positioning, regular
skin care, and the new therapeutic, undulating beds, pressure sores
will occur in immobilized people. But some occur because a patient is
debilitated, septic, undernourished, or has poor circulation. Healing
depends as much on a patient's health as on a nurse's technique.)

"These days, how are you doing?"

"Usually four out of six Timbits." He grinned.

"Ahh, Timbit scores." Again, not funny, but we laughed. Then I asked him a question that's no laughing matter. "What has all this done to your marriage?"

"Veronique accepts it more than me. 'I'd rather have you this way than not at all,' she says. Her folks were worried because at first she planned to quit her job and stay home to take care of me, but we both knew it would ruin our marriage. Besides, we need her income. Having the nurses come in every morning and evening makes it possible for her to get back to work and have a break from caregiving. Luckily, my injury is severe enough to qualify for twice-daily nursing visits," he says with a rueful smirk at his stroke of "luck."

Silence falls and I try to gauge if he's tiring of my questions. Maybe I should get going and let him and Rhonda get on with his day. I thanked him for his time and put my pen and notebook away.

"I'm glad to be of help," Gaétan said. "You can ask me anything." He flashes his full, animated smile that contrasts so sharply with his prone, still body. "Absolutely anything."

Do I dare ask him what comes to mind as I sit here on their bed, the intimate smell of sleep still lingering in the air? I look at a photograph of his wife hanging on the wall on his side of the bed. She's beautiful, her toned body draped only in a diaphanous scarf.

"Anything?" I ask.

"Of course."

Okay. Here goes. "Sex. How do you have sex?"

He gave an easygoing chuckle. "I'd like to tell you about that. I don't get erect, so we can't have intercourse, but Veronique sits on top of me and I give her oral sex. I've gotten good at it. That's what she says, anyway."

"How about you?" How to say this . . . "How do you get . . . pleasure?"

"Viagra didn't work for me, but I may get an implant. There are some new treatments, including surgery, I'd like to try that might make me hard."

"Why go to the trouble if you can't feel it, anyway?"

"It would be for her, to feel me inside her. For me, too, to know that I'm inside her. For me now, sex is all about giving. Veronique's arousal turns me on, so I try to give her as many orgasms as I can. I have to say, she's a very willing participant."

"But when she kisses you or touches you . . . you can't feel that? Not at all?"

"I imagine how it feels, I remember how it felt. No, I can't have an orgasm, but I'm coming to terms with that – excuse the bad pun. Giving pleasure to her is what turns me on now. I'd like to be able to have intercourse, but even though I won't feel it, I'll *know* it."

"Were you always so comfortable talking about your sex life?"

"No, not at all, but the nurses have helped me. Especially Rhonda. We talk about it all the time. There's nothing I can't say to Rhonda." She looks up from disposing of the dressing change equipment and she and Gaétan exchange another glance of understanding.

"But tell me, when you have a urine bag on your abdomen and a pressure sore on your butt, how do you get into the mood?"

"Sex takes place in my mind, but it definitely has to be planned. We can't be spontaneous because Veronique has to use the lifter to get me on the bed. I guess that's our foreplay."

I looked at the swinging bar of the lifter that he holds on to. For a moment, it looks like what a trapeze artist would use. "Is that all you use the lifter for?"

"What kinky purpose were you thinking of?"

"You read my mind!" The three of us laughed at that.

I went out of the room while Rhonda got Gaétan up into his electric wheelchair. Sure, I could have stayed while she did that, but I wanted to give him back some privacy. Thinking it over now, I realize I also chose to leave the room to protect myself from the heartbreaking sight of this proud, handsome, virile man suspended helplessly in the air, folded into the stained hammock of the hydraulic lifter device.

Out in the sunny kitchen, I made a full pot of coffee. Gaétan rolled in with Rhonda beside him. I'm sure that sitting upright, meeting me eye to eye, must feel more dignified, than talking to me lying down while I'm sitting up. We chatted for a few minutes about our kids and music we like. We admired the view from his window of a beautiful lake that's practically outside his doorstep, just a short distance from this house to the shore.

Gaétan's story is tragic, but I didn't feel sadness or pity – he's not the least bit pitiful. A tragedy demands that one choose life, and I feel he has done that. He'll make his new life. He's on his way. This man is healthy. He's not sick, just broken, and well on the mend. He plans to go back to work in two weeks for a few hours a day to ease back into it, and he's looking forward to that. "Not as much for the income as an opportunity to think of things other than my situation."

"Are you still okay sharing your story with others?" I did a hasty, cursory assessment of his emotions as I put on my coat. He seemed fine, but I wondered if it made him feel vulnerable to open up to a complete stranger who suddenly leaves, taking off with a piece of his story to share with the world.

"I'm okay," he assured me. "I'm happy to do what I can for VON. Anything for the nurses."

I bent down to hug him goodbye and felt how much he wanted to hug me back, and his frustration at not being able to do that. I hoped he felt the warmth I felt for him, but what about the warmth of my body against his chest? Can he feel my beating heart against his beating heart? Does he have any sensation whatsoever of my arms around him, embracing him tightly? No, he does not. I know the anatomy and physiology of a spinal cord break. But, maybe there are times when *knowing* is as good as *feeling*. If so, he feels my hug in the way that a hug matters most.

18

HOME AT LAST

BACK HOME, I unpacked and relaxed. I did a few shifts in the ICU, and then, a few days later, repacked and set out on my next trip. Of course, I picked up a stack of letters from Audrey that had arrived while I was gone. But these ones I dreaded opening because I knew I had disappointed her by missing her party. I can feel the reproach in her letters – the teddy bear, kitten, valentine, and snowflake decorations notwithstanding.

> I was crushed and broken-hearted not to see you at my party. I started to cry but as the Guest of Honour, I had to keep up a brave face. However, I thank you for your recent and properly dated letter of birthday greetings. I also appreciated your telephone call on my birthday, but not the frustration I heard in your voice with my hearing difficulties. . . . Please be more patient with me as I am old.

> My party was a big hit. You missed a great event. I was the talk of the town. Everyone was there. My friends and all the local "who's who," including the mayor. No flowers, of course. My eulogy was

read splendidly by our minister, Reverend Matthew Kydd. Here
are newspaper clippings about the event of the season.

. . . still trying to cope with the tortuous toilet seat. . . . I'm deteriorating fast. My back is going downhill, my vision is failing
frightfully fast, and my hearing is hilarious. Make your own diagnosis. . . . I'm glad I got to see you while I was still partly alive.

. . . thank you for your powerful letter, a mini-sermonette it was,
really. Enough preaching about flu shots and taking care of myself.
Come visit me before it's too late. . . . It is a chaotic life you lead
with all of this travelling from pillar to post and to'ing and fro'ing
all over the country. Is it safe for your heart to carry on like this? A
visit to precious, peaceful Kemptville is the rest cure you need.

Right now, I'm driving westward along this stretch of highway to
London, the exact opposite direction from Kemptville. This strip of
highway between Toronto and Windsor, with London midway, is
notorious for the highest rate of motor vehicle accidents in Canada. It
is a monotonous stretch with few rest stops to break the tedium.
Driving at an average clip, it takes three and a half hours to get to
Windsor, but I'm driving only halfway, to London. I'm a confident
driver, not the least bit nervous, even now in winter with unexpected
flurries and snow squalls that can kick up at a moment's notice or the
black ice that you can't see but sure can feel when you slide into it.

Tomorrow morning I have a meeting with a man named Wayne
Ranta. Once homeless, he now lives in government-subsidized housing. The VON office didn't tell me any more than that.

"Look at me. I'm down to 120. Skin and bones," Wayne says. "I grew up
on the farm, milked cows, had a mother who fed me well. When I left
home I was a strapping 190, all muscle. I had nineteen-inch arms,
forty-four waist. I don't want to brag or nothin' . . ."

We're sitting in Wayne's one-bedroom apartment — well, I'm the
one sitting. He's crouching, because there is no other folding chair but
this one. When I arrived, Wayne offered me the chair. "But you should
be the one to sit," I said. No, he insisted I take the chair. He won
because he promised if he gets tired he'll rest on his scooter, which is
parked in the corner of the empty, echo-y room. Wayne probably does
prefer to crouch. Because of his chronic obstructive pulmonary disease (COPD) — and, in his case, that means emphysema, bronchitis,
and a recent bout of pneumonia — crouching on the floor is probably
more comfortable. This position likely eases his breathing. Many
patients with COPD use this manoeuvre because the physiological
mechanism behind it is real. Compressing the diaphragm increases
the body's natural "PEEP," the positive end-tidal expiratory pressure
in his lungs, thereby easing the work of breathing.

We sit together in this dim space, lit by only a yellow light bulb
hanging from the ceiling, bare and cheerless — but Wayne is pleased,
even proud of it. He's fifty-four. That's my age, too, but I *look* fifty-four;
Wayne looks seventy. Unshaven, bent over, with shaggy grey hair that
makes me think he trimmed it himself with a pair of dull shears, he's
an old man in baggy jeans, a faded plaid shirt, and a pair of crocheted
maroon slippers made by a VON volunteer. Wayne has the barrel chest
and clubbed fingers distinctive of COPD patients, a gaunt frame, and
long, nicotine-stained fingers. Looking around, I see that furni-
ture-wise, there's not much, only a bed, a TV, and the one folding chair
that I'm currently occupying.

"VON tried to give me a used couch, but they'd already given me a
winter coat, so I told them to give the couch to someone else."

We've only been chatting for a few minutes, but speaking is hard work
for Wayne. His breathing is already laboured. My instinct urges me to
suggest he stop talking to conserve his energy but he desperately wants
to speak. He's grateful to VON and wants to give back by telling his story.

When he was ready to be discharged from the hospital, Wayne had
no way of getting home, so a VON program called Home at Last sent an

attendant to pick him up, get him groceries, and fill his prescriptions. The attendant made sure the heat was on and checked that Wayne had a sufficient supply of oxygen tanks. "The guy even stayed and made me a cup of tea. I don't drink tea, only coffee, but it's the thought that counts, eh? It's a lot better than coming home like last time by myself to a cold room in the men's shelter."

Luckily, a home care nurse visited Wayne for the next few days to help prevent a readmission to the hospital.

"I sure didn't want to go back there and I didn't want to go to the family doctor I'd been seeing either. She'd been threatening to fire me if I didn't do what she said." He stops to catch his breath. "So, I wrote her a diplomatic letter to say I was firing *her*. I didn't like her attitude." He stops for another breath. "My lungs are shot. Now, my kidneys are acting up."

"Did you have this place to come to after your hospital stay?" I ask, drawing out my words so as to give him more time to catch his breath before continuing his story.

He shakes his head now. He breathes.

"You must have been living in another place before this one . . ."

I wait for a few moments. "So, I guess you were in another place before this one?"

"I was living in a rusted out car," he says, and seems ready to continue. "It was a helluva lot better than a park bench. I found it parked on a dead end, in an alley . . . and that's where I lived until I got pneumonia. Then I had no choice but to go into the hospital. That was in December, right before Christmas."

"So, you knew it was pneumonia?"

"Yup. I've had it so many times before. Each time I need antibiotics. The IV ones. I tried to tell them that, but they gave me the pills instead. But . . . I know they don't work for me. They just wouldn't listen and, sure enough, I had to go back a few days later. They said that to give me IV antibiotics, they'd have to admit me. 'Okay, admit me,' I said, and the doctor told me — this is word for word what he said: 'In order to get . . . admitted to the hospital you have to have an address.'

He thought I was trying to use the hospital for a place to stay, but I was seriously sick, man. 'I have pneumonia,' I said, but he said it was only a cold. 'The tablets you gave me aren't working. I'm getting worse.' 'We'll give you different ones,' he said and walked away. After two more visits to the ER, each time in worse shape, I got admitted on the fifth one and ended up having to stay there for seven weeks. I just got out a few days ago. I've had bad experiences with doctors. You get the odd one who's down-to-earth but some think they're God."

Wayne goes on to tell me about other hospitalizations and his many chronic medical problems such as high blood pressure, a long-standing abscessed vein that still hasn't healed, and more.

"Yes, I was an IV drug user. I admit it. But I'm clean now . . ."

As Wayne tells me about his drug abuse history and multiple medical issues, I start to do something a nurse should never do. I let my attention drift away. I allow my mind to wander from what Wayne is saying. I look around the room. Old newspapers are taped over the windows to keep out the light. A pack of cigarettes is hidden under a TV guide and there's an ashtray on top of the television. Along the window ledge is a scattering of pennies and a few respiratory inhalers.

Wayne is still talking. I make an effort to listen, but I can't. I want to ask him about something else. So I do another thing a nurse should never do. I interrupt him.

"Wayne, tell me. How did it happen that you ended up like this?"

He smiles sadly. "It's quite a story. Do you want to hear it?"

Of course I do, and he wants to tell me.

"I had a good upbringing, even played hockey."

"No better upbringing than that," I agree.

"Yup. And I was a good hockey player. Then I became an expert in electronics. I got married, had three houses, all paid . . . up. Then I got . . . a sleep disorder. They told me I was getting no REM sleep. You're supposed . . . to have 25 per cent REM, but I had only 3 per cent, so I was always tired." He stops to adjust his oxygen regulator and reposition his nasal prongs to make them more comfortable in his nostrils. "I . . . was an electronics expert – did I mention that? I built a radio transmitter at age seven. Electronics was my hobby and became my work. My businesses were eating up the cash. I lost all . . . my money. My wife complained I was never home. I lost hold of my sanity. Spent two years trying to get it back. I had a breakdown. I developed a sleeping disorder. It all fell apart and I was out of work . . . I left everything to the wife. I became Oscar the Grouch. I developed an obsessive-compulsive disorder and would only eat food that . . . came in cans. I had three . . . kids, but it might actually be more like four or five out there somewhere. I could fix anything – TVs, VCRs, computers . . . . Up until then, I was making six hundred dollars a week – take home. It was around this time that the government . . . came out with a law that when you turned the key in the car the headlights had to come on. It was a safety thing. Yup, it was an idea adopted from Sweden. They also legislated mandatory seat belts, too. . . . Now we all have to use seat belts, right? I was just about to go into the Stop'n'Go coffee business. Tim Hortons wasn't around at the time. Then they came out with this new law. . . . I figured out how to do it and steered all my capital into making a prototype. It was a device connected to the ignition that would automatically switch on the lights. I was working night and day on it, never sleeping."

Reluctantly, Wayne stops to turn up the flow on his oxygen tank There's only a half a tank left, so I go over to the stacked cylinders in the hallway entrance. I hoist one up and bring it over. *These things are heavy for me. How does he manage to haul them over and reconnect them to the tank?*

Wayne's jumbled story is easy to piece together, and his obvious intelligence and genuine humility touch me deeply. I am on his side, rooting for him.

"So, you were working on your invention, day and night, and living on your own?"

"Nope. By then I was living in a shelter, a mission for . . . men. I found a wonderful doctor who diagnosed me with a heart arrhythmia. She ordered some test and while they were doing it, they all left me alone . . .

in a room . . . for a long time. I was sure I was going to die. That was the
scariest thing in my life. *Ever.* I freaked out and they had to sedate me and
I don't know what happened after then. Yesterday, I had to go back in to
see an eye doctor and I was worried they'd do that test again. I keep reliving it in my mind, but it didn't happen again. And sure, enough, ol' VON
brought me home again after my appointment."

"So, the lights had to come on when you turned on the car?" I prompt,
rushing him along – again, not recommended – but I want to know how
this story turns out before he runs out of steam.

"Oh, yeah, so my father . . . had been bugging me for months to
invest in this thing that would turn the lights on when you start up the
car. 'Wayne, you can make one of these,' he said. Sure, I could. I went
to Radio Shack, bought some junk . . . and built a prototype. I took it to
one of the big Japanese carmakers. As soon as they saw it, they loved
it. 'We'll manufacture it and sell it,' they said. I took all my money out
of the coffee shop – $200,000 – and got government approvals up the
ying yang . . . went back to them, made a hundred prototypes at a hundred dollars a piece to test out in their cars. Man, I worked twenty-four
hours a day to get 'em done. You know what? They liked it so much the
bastards took my design and ran with it. Never heard from them again.
Now, as you know, the headlights come on whenever you turn on a car."

There was a Hollywood movie similar to this, I tell him. It's about
the guy who invented intermittent windshield wipers. His idea was
stolen, but he went after the big automakers in Detroit. It took a big
fight and a lawsuit, but he ended up getting compensation.

"I haven't had the time to go after them."

Sadly, Wayne needs more than time – he needs wherewithal, energy,
and health to just stay alive. Whether or not Wayne's story is verifiable
or merely a "reality show in his own mind" doesn't matter to me. Right
now, Wayne is exhausted. He can't do anything but breathe.

And yet, there's more he wants to say.

"So I never heard back from them. All my hard work and my life
savings – gone. Eventually, I picked myself up and learned computer

coding, even mastered five programming languages. Then my mother died. A month later, my father remarried. He's a piece of work, that guy. Now I have no contact with my family. I don't fit in. I guess you could say I'm the black sheep. My grandmother hated me. She'd buy my sisters a toy, but nothing for me." His face shows this old hurt as if it happened recently, not years ago. "I guess you could say I'm a loser. A lost cause."

"No, Wayne, you are a *found* cause. I think you're a genius."

"Yeah, a genius of self-destruction." He looks down at the ground and then over at the box of cigarettes. "Yeah, I'd say I'm smarter than the average bear . . ."

He's well into his second tank of oxygen and motions for me to bring a third from the hallway. I can't stay to the end of the second cylinder, but he wants it nearby, close at hand.

He looks up at me from where he's still crouching on the floor, learning slightly forward. "Next question, please."

"What do you do to occupy your time?"

"Watch TV."

"Are you lonely?"

"Yes, but I have to stay indoors . . . so my lungs'll heal."

"What about friends?"

"I limit my friendships . . . I've lost track of a lot of people. . . . So many people let me down, stole my money. A VON lady calls every day to check on me. They send a nice lady once a week to help me shower. I can't do it by myself. I've got a scooter so I can get groceries."

"Do you cook for yourself? What do you eat?"

He nods over at the fridge and I get up to have a look. A half a loaf of bread, a few bottles of beer, and an open can of baked beans, the jagged lid sticking out. I look around the tiny kitchenette. On the countertop is a small, dented pot, resting upside down on a threadbare rag. The site of that lone, tin pot makes me unspeakably sad.

"They got me Meals on Wheels," Wayne says to explain why there's so little in his fridge. "I make each one last for two meals."

"Are they that expensive?"

"No, but I am saving up for new shoes. My disability cheques cover my needs. On Tuesday mornings there's a communal lunch in this building for two dollars. Free coffee and doughnuts from Timmie's on Monday mornings. The government got me the scooter. There's a drop-in centre where I go on the Internet. When I'm feeling better, I want go over there and help other homeless guys. I've been there and now I have a home. I want them to see it's possible."

He has to choose between eating and walking? That is so wrong. I know what I'll do. I'll take him home with me. Feed him soup. Build him up. Let him enjoy our comfortable home. He can live in our basement, I'm sure my family won't mind . . .

Wayne sees I'm sad and tries to cheer me up. "Don't worry about me. This is the best home I've ever had." He smiles not just for my benefit but also because he's truly content. I can see that. Even if my madcap scheme were feasible, I feel certain Wayne would turn it down. He doesn't want to live with me and my family. He wants to live here. This is his home. He's at home here. Home at last.

I drive on along the remaining stretch of this treacherous highway on my way to Windsor. Got to make it there tonight, check into the hotel, get a good night's sleep. Tomorrow, I have an early morning visit booked. It's dark and I'm sleepy, but thinking about Wayne's story keeps me awake. It's easy to see how incredibly easy it would be to end up alone and homeless. One setback in life can lead to another and another, in a rapid downward spiral; it could happen to anyone.

As I drive along, I carry a heaviness that I can't shake off. I keep reminding myself to concentrate on the road ahead. I flip the radio stations from CBC evening news to Adele to Mozart to Kanye. It surprises me how upset I feel. How can this be? I'm an old hardened hospital nurse, aren't I? I should be able to handle my emotions after all these years.

Yes, I've learned the tricks of the trade. How could I have worked in the ICU so long if every sad thing that came along affected me? Nurses know how to lighten the load with jokes, banter, and gossip. Another tried-and-true method is to *keep busy*. That's easy because there's always so much to *do*. There are some shifts when we don't have a moment to sit for the entire twelve hours. Another thing that helps is the magical delusion that the drastic things that happen to our patients won't happen to us or someone we love. And we read only a single, isolated page from the hundreds of chapters of the entire novel of a person's life. That minimizes our exposure. It allows us to focus on the numbers and machines, the liver and kidneys, the cells and molecules – no pesky emotions there.

But it's infuriating that there are hungry people in our wealthy country. I have eaten super-sized meals, thrown out leftovers, carried home doggy bags from restaurant meals. I've even thrown out food if it's stale or wilted, or if my refrigerator is too crowded, just to free up space so I can buy more food. But I try to stay focused on my anger at the world's injustices rather than my sadness about Wayne. Anger keeps me alert, better for driving alone on this cold, dark highway.

19

LA DOLCE VITA

ALL I CAN SAY IS, when I get old and infirm, either shoot me or put me in a place like this.

This is "La Dolce Vita," once an elegant, rustic Italian trattoria that has been revamped and turned into an elegant, rustic retirement home. It is for long-term residents who are independent, but five beds are reserved for people who need a shorter-term stay and some nursing care. It's exactly what Geriatric Emergency Manager Magda said was needed – "crisis placement" for elders who need a supportive transition until they're ready to go home.

I meet Ethel, a senior here to recover after a bad fall at home. She'll stay until she, well, gets back on her feet. She's part of DETOUR: Deterring Emergency Time Offering Urgent Respite. It's a stopgap remedy, a bridge to home, and Ethel looks like she's well on her way.

For elders, falls are a big deal. They are so common yet so preventable; they can happen so easily, but recovery can take months. It can be a simple tumble that can initiate a whole chain reaction of decline and a lengthy hospitalization. I've seen it myself, but from the other end, when it's far too late to intervene.

We sit in Ethel's nicely furnished room to chat. She's wearing a bright coral blouse and white pants, makeup nicely done. She's put aside her crocheting so she can test her blood sugar with her glucometer. Ethel has no difficulty doing that and, at the same time, recounting the story of how she landed up in this place that, as nice as it is, is not her *home*.

"I had just gotten out of the shower when I slipped and fell. I didn't have my lifeline on me. I lay there on the bathroom floor. Lost my urine three times – *sooo* embarrassing – my poor cat stood over me, nudging me like, *Mommy get up, I want my breakfast.*" Trust a cat! "I heard the sound of my bone cracking when down I went." She sees the result of her blood sugar test and decides on the dosage of her pre-lunch insulin. "I inched my way along the floor to the phone, dozing off from time to time. Ting Ling kept meowing to wake me up. He knew something was wrong with Mommy. People don't give animals enough credit. It took me two days to get to the phone. I called 911. I was okay but Ting Ling was real mad. He was hungry. My tailbone was cracked and I had a concussion – from a good whack on the head – and my arm was bruised. They kept me overnight in the hospital, but I couldn't go home. So they brought me here to get my strength back." Ethel draws up the insulin, raises her pant leg, and gives herself the shot in her thigh.

With her lively face, busy hands – manicured in the exact same shade of coral as her blouse – I can see that Ethel, a retired accountant, a bridge and mah-jong player, is content.

"It's so nice here, would you like to stay?"

"No way! I'm not ready for this place. I want to get back home. This is just a temporary fix to get me back on my feet.

"But I do like it here. They check on me throughout the day. Once, I was on the toilet and they knocked, didn't hear me answer and came right in. It was embarrassing, but worth it for the security of knowing they are there." Ethel picks up her afghan-in-progress and continues. "Coincidentally, I found my husband on the floor. Five years in a row he had a heart attack. Every fall he had a fall. He died. We'd been going to Daytona Beach for twenty years, but always made sure to return to Canada for a few months to keep our health insurance. He was my second

husband. My first used his hands on me, so I got rid of him. I didn't have
health care in Florida, so I had to sell the house and come back. I have a
nice apartment here and I'm looking forward to getting back to it."

"What's it been like to be here for the past few weeks?" I ask.

"I love it here. It's so clean. It even smells clean – pine and lemony.
The homey Italian cooking is dee-licious. My fall changed everything. I
couldn't take care of myself. But I can now. I'm almost ready to go home.
But first, let's go have lunch. Yippee! It's Eggplant Parmigiana day!"

After lunch, I drive to VON's Chronic Pain Management Clinic to learn
more about the "good life" from Nurse Stephanie Vandevenne. She's
the manager of the team that consists of a nurse practitioner, doctor,
social worker, physiotherapist, and occupational therapist. They see
clients with complex pain issues such as back pain, sciatica, or fibromyalgia, and often visit them at home to obtain a detailed history of
their problem and how they are managing.

As for fibromyalgia, it's a diagnosis that isn't given much credence
in my hospital world because no precise etiology or pathology has ever
been discovered. However, here it is taken very seriously.

"The pain is real to the person suffering," Stephanie says. "It can be
whole body pain, often initiated by a trauma. Whether it's emotional or
physical, it's pain. In many cases of fibromyalgia there is a past history
of sexual abuse. When they finally come to us they have tried many
things and have been pushing themselves to cope as best as they can."

Clients that come to this clinic usually bring a long list of medications that they are living on, just trying to cope with their pain. "We
work with them to provide better management of their meds and
expand their repertoire of modalities they can use to manage their
pain." She quotes the old adage we all learn in doctor or nurse school
but find difficult to practise: "Pain is whatever the person says it is."
In the hospital, it has often been more like "pain is what we can see and
measure, and we are the ones in control of its treatment," but there's
definitely change afoot to partnerships with patients. Stephanie and

the Pain Clinic team use videoconferencing because clients aren't always feeling well enough to come in. In fact, the two clients she asked to come today to talk with me are going to phone it in. They both cancelled because they weren't feeling well.

Dixie is a construction worker who misses her job. She hasn't been able to work for the past two years due to constant pain from a work-related injury. "I hate not working but I'm making progress. I can now bend down to put on a pair of jeans and withstand the pressure of the denim on my back – that's a huge achievement. I go to water therapy classes in a heated pool and have cut back on my meds. I hate them. Today, the pain woke me up, like an electric shock. I did hard physical work for fifteen years and had occasional aches and pains, but nothing like this. A lot of people in chronic pain don't help themselves but I'm not like that. I take as few narcotics as possible. The pain team taught me to trust my instinct and do what works for me. They give me a lot of support, understanding, and information. One way or another, I'm going to beat this thing."

I wasn't expecting such an upbeat, inspiring story about pain.

Next up is Connie. She gives me the "Reader's Digest version," the abridged nutshell of her pain story. "Single mom. Oncology nurse. Breast cancer. Chemo. Radiation. Now, constant bone and back pain. There were no bone metastases on my scans, so 'there's no reason you should be in pain,' my doctor said, but let me tell you, I was in pain. Did she think I was faking it? But here, these people don't write me off as crazy or looking for drugs. 'This is not in your head,' this pain clinic doctor said. 'Your pain is real. It's peripheral neuropathy related to the chemo. That won't show up on a scan.' Here, I get a sense of genuine compassion and empathy. I've been to hell and back, yet when I walk into this clinic and meet people with genuine compassion, it makes me feel I'm not alone. These people are on my side. It's a partnership. They've given me more to add to my tool box for coping with this thing. They gave me options, rather than sitting here feeling hopeless. My pain is seven out of ten most days. Today it's nine out of ten. It's a rough day, that's why I couldn't come in to meet you in person. But I always say, if you're crying into your beer, you're just watering it down, and I don't want to that, do I?"

I met Nurse Manager Andrew Ward back at the AGM, and seeing him again today I remember his fast-pace tempo and trademark high-energy passion for his work at VON. He's committed to bringing healthy breakfasts to school kids. It's obviously a real need; for some of these children, this meal is their only secure source of food.

"The program is for everyone, not just poor kids. It levels the playing field, eliminates stigma. There's more participation if no one is singled out. There's no reason anyone should be hungry in this country. Research has shown that it takes twelve tries for a kid to get used to a new food, but if they eat with peers, it takes only four exposures. Accessing healthy food is not just about poverty, it's about mental health, too. Grandmothers cooking in the kitchen? Sitting down to eat a meal as a family? Those days are long gone. We bring in fruits and vegetables from local farms. We want every child to have the opportunity to have a healthy meal to start the day. We need to get away from the fast-food thinking around food."

A few months ago, I would have wondered what nutrition or children's breakfasts had to do with nursing. Now I know that they have everything to do with nursing; these are pure nursing concerns.

If I didn't know that Liz Mikol was a nurse, the sight of her umbrella hanging from an IV pole in the corner of her office would be a tip-off. That is such a nurse thing to do – unexpectedly playful and creatively practical – and Liz is *sooo* nurse. With her take-charge, go-to, can-do attitude, she's the nurse manager of the nursing station on Pelee Island, just off the shore of Lake Erie, where emergency services can be reached only by ferry, helicopter, or plane. Liz speaks in short bursts that have the staccato rhythm of a checklist, like the ones pilots use. Her mind is quick but so organized that it's easy to follow her.

"They called me. On a Saturday. 'Open the nursing station on Monday,' they told me. And I did. Before that, I'd done everything as a nurse. Oncology? Check. General medicine? Check. ER? Check. ICU? Check. But primary care? No thank you. Not interested."

"That was my reaction, too. At first."

Liz nods in agreement. "I'm a very fast-paced person. Didn't think I'd like it. Was reluctant at first. Now, I love it. It's a different type of nursing. For sure. You get to know your patients. They depend on you. You're out there on your own. It's all up to you. I like to work hard – seven days a week. Then I discovered Pelee Island. It's exactly like the TV show *Corner Gas*. Everyone knows each other and is involved in each other's lives. In a good way.

"My husband is a nurse, too. We get to the island by ferry or a twenty-minute flight in a small plane. It depends if there's weather. We are only around two hundred, but in the summer, the population swells to thousands. We have an inordinate amount of motor vehicle accidents, most due to driving under the influence. It's a huge problem, especially in the summer. I've taken a suture course and we're well stocked with antibiotics, epinephrine for anaphylaxis, and tetanus vaccine. Once, two girls were in a car accident. One broke her sternum. Huge risk of puncture to the heart or the lungs. The weather was bad. We couldn't bring them in. Videoconferencing with a camera and a stethoscope to an ED doctor in Windsor, plus IV fluid resuscitation, back boards, and neck braces, kept them stable until the weather cleared and we could transfer them to Windsor. If they'd been bleeding we'd've had to call the air force at Trenton to chopper them in. Those girls are just fine now. The nursing station can be busy, but that's okay, because I'm a go-go-go type."

"I see that." I can hardly keep up with her. Luckily, I write fast.

"One thing – I don't like snakes. There are a lot of snakes on the island. All harmless, but *still*. You have to be a nature lover to come here. I'm not. I'm a city girl. I'm not a hiker, not a biker, not a birder. What I like is people. The people on Pelee Island are the warmest, kindest people you'll ever meet. It's a real community. I'm a Toronto girl, so it's different for me. On the island, they go out of their way to help you. They love the nursing station. They made us king and queen and put us on a boat around the island. It's like family. In the winter, nothing is open. There are lots of coyote, deer, birdwatchers. We have a sanctuary here for migratory birds. In the summer we get a lot of American tourists. Artists and writers, even Margaret Atwood has a place on the island. There are turtles, snakes. Police only in the summer, not the rest of the year, and we even have a winery."

She hardly stops for a breath and I can't stop my note-taking, even for a moment. There seem to be a lot of high-energy, fast-talking people at VON.

"'You must be kidding,' I said when Frank suggested we move there, but he fell in love with the place and then I did, too. We are so close to the people on the island. Neighbourhood parties? Potlucks? I never experienced that in Toronto. Here, people rely on each other, help each other, the doors are open. Most people in Toronto don't even know their neighbours. My husband was cutting wood. A neighbour came to help. It's the Pelee way. It's something unique and you want to be a part of that. There's a homeless man who lives in a shack with holes in the ceiling. There are hundreds of cats and he hoards paper bags. People invite him into their homes, where he showers and has a meal. We all look after him. Where else do you find this? Anywhere else, they'd have condemned the house. Written him off. We bought a house on the lake. It would cost a few million dollars in Toronto. In their wildest dreams they never thought they'd get a nursing couple to stay on the island. It's great for them and for us. Yes, it's a sweet life."

20

BUTTERFLIES AND BALLOONS

"PEOPLE HAVE A NEED TO CREATE rituals that are meaningful to them," Auedrah DeHeus says. She works with the Kids' Circle, a support group for children with a loved one who's dying and for children grieving a loved one who has died.

"Unfortunately, it was a string of copy-cat teen suicides that got this program off the ground. Every time there's a tragedy in the community, there is an upsurge in need for more groups like this."

They hold a butterfly release event. (It used to be a balloon release until it was discovered that birds got caught in the deflated balloons or choked on them.) The butterflies are donated by the local nursery, and a ceremony is held where the kids open the box and allow their butterfly to fly away. In another event, the kids make T-shirts with pictures of their loved one on them and decorate them; they create memory boxes and garden stones of remembrance.

Auedrah believes we need new rituals like these because a lot of people don't believe in organized religion the way they used to, yet are still searching for spiritual expression.

"Most children believe in heaven," she says, "but that seems to change as they get older. When it comes to dealing with death, many turn to God or some sort of spirit that gives them hope that their loved one is around all the time."

She tells of a young Ojibway woman who was grieving the loss of her sister, whose name meant *sweet, flowing water*.

"She was cynical yet kept coming to the group," Auedrah says. "The day we released balloons filled with helium, she followed her balloon, which eventually landed in a stream. That was a very meaningful moment to her, especially considering her dead sister's name. Somehow that helped bring her some peace."

Auedrah tells me of a teen who was bullied at school. When his dad died, his peers said things like, "Your dad died because you're stupid." The boy told only Auedrah about his plan to kill himself. He even mentioned a rope he'd hidden behind some hockey sticks in the garage. Auedrah called his mother and asked her, "Are there ropes in a box behind the hockey sticks in the garage?" There were. Together they took her son to the hospital and stayed with him there.

"And yes, I do attend deaths in people's homes and even some funerals," Auedrah says. "They always tell us not to get attached, don't they? But how can you not? And why shouldn't we get attached? If we lose that genuine compassion that VON is known for, that we pride ourselves on offering, then who are we? I love becoming attached to my clients. It adds so much to my life."

Originally, the program was kept secret to protect the children's privacy, but that only reinforced the stigma of death. Bringing it out of the closet became more important than keeping it on the down low, under wraps.

"Most people want to share their stories, not keep them to themselves, don't you find?"

Yes, I agree. Most people are longing to tell their stories. In fact, they're *desperate* to share their stories with someone who will listen and acknowledge their experience. More people want to be seen and known than anonymous or forgotten. In fact, many people write to tell me they have a book inside them. I encourage them to write it. "What's the point?" they often ask. Do it for yourself, I tell them. Or write it for your family, your friends.

To learn more about stories, I visit Nurse Jane Parr in her office in the Kids' Circle building. Jane trains volunteers to visit people who have life-threatening conditions and help them record their life story, or write letters, or create a scrapbook or video for those they are leaving behind. She suggests questions to cue people, to spark memory and conversation. Documented in the person's handwriting, the lost art of storytelling in the person's own words – it's such a comfort to those left behind.

"Our society is so different nowadays," Jane laments. "People keep to themselves and keep themselves private. Neighbours don't even know each other. Helping connections used to spring up naturally within a community without formal organization, but it doesn't always happen like that anymore. Families are often spread out over the globe, people don't want to interfere with others, or they don't know how to help."

I return to the room where Auedrah holds the Kids' Circle sessions and I sit on the child-sized chairs and read the permanent-ink messages written on the pink, green, and yellow rubber, interlocking tiles:

I hope you are having fun up in heaven.

Sorry for what happened. Love, Me.

You are with MJ reads another message with a hand-drawn picture of Michael Jackson standing with the artist's father in heaven.

I wish I had died with you. Then we could be together.

I look up from reading the tiles to meet Helena Walls, who has just walked in. Helena's husband died two years ago and despite her own grief at this fairly recent loss, she's here to tell me about her children's grief and their road to healing. They were her greatest worry, especially since two of them witnessed their father's death.

"Each of my three children know when I'm having a bad day and they are very kind to me." Helena dabs at her eyes with a tissue, then puts it into her purse as if to say there will be no more crying – at least not today.

"Today is a good day and I'm happy to talk with you," she says.

That's good, because I was feeling worried about having Helena relive her tragedy, but no, she says, she wanted to come in to talk with me. She hopes that sharing her story will help others, as others' stories have helped her.

"Aaron was so full of energy, so vital. He'd gone off to the marina with my two older girls to check on the boat. My son, who was still a baby, stayed home with me. A few hours later, when two police officers showed up at my door, I thought nothing of it. 'There's been a boating accident,' they told me. 'What does this have to do with me?' I thought. 'At the marina,' they said, and then it hit me."

Only later was Helena able to piece together what happened. Their eight-year-old daughter had been swimming, wearing a life jacket that was attached to a rope tied to the dock. Suddenly, the rope loosened and let go. "She was beginning to float away and wasn't able to get back to the dock. With no hesitation, Aaron dove into the water to save her. He managed to get our daughter to safety, but he couldn't make it back himself. We don't know why. He was an excellent swimmer. But the two girls stood on the dock and watched their father drown. They were devastated."

The two sisters withdrew, wouldn't talk to anyone. "They became empty shells of their sweet, innocent selves. They had been such happy children before the accident. They had lots of friends, loved to laugh and play with their friends, but now, they stopped talking, stopped smiling. They blamed themselves for what had happened. The older one had flashbacks every time she heard the sound of running water, even the sound of the shower, or toilet. They used to love swimming but were now traumatized around anything to do with water.

"I didn't know how to help them. Then we met Auedrah, here at the Kids' Circle. They would only talk to her. She showed them that nothing they could have done would have made the outcome any different. Their dad did what any dad would do – save his child – and he doesn't blame them. His kids were everything to him. Auedrah helped them let go of their guilt. She saved the girls' emotional and mental health. Here, they could grieve with other kids who know what they are going through. They are completely back to themselves, enjoying life again. They are both good swimmers and love the water. They now remember their father as the incredible, fun dad he was, and not only the horrible circumstances of his death."

She points to one of the pink tiles. That's her daughter's handwriting.

I miss you tucking me in at night, Daddy. You were my best friend.

I'm meeting Jackie Wells for lunch, but maybe I should grab a snack beforehand? Judging by my last encounter with Jackie – last June at the annual general meeting – there'll be no eating. With Jackie, all I can do is listen and think, not cut up food, lift a fork, chew, and swallow.

"Hellooooo, there!" She arrives in the restaurant, suddenly appearing in front of me, as if out of nowhere, and wraps me in a tight hug. Here again are those bright blue eyes, tight curls, that vivacious presence. We sit opposite each other in a booth, to chat and – hopefully – eat lunch. I want to have my say first.

"I gotta tell you, Jackie, when we first met, I had no idea what you were talking about. 'Home care.' 'Community supports.' I couldn't picture it. I thought nursing was taking care of sick people. I thought health care was the hospital. After all, I've spent thirty years of my life working in hospitals." A fact that now makes me think, *Look at all I have missed out on.*

"Health care is not doctors and medical procedures," Jackie jumps in. "Nor is it hospitals, where the focus is disease and diagnosis. Do they ever look at the person? Do they even get to know the person?"

"But how can we? Who has time to get to know people?" I say, getting a word or two in edgewise. "Some nurses say getting to know the patient makes it harder to care for them."

"I would challenge that," Jackie says, and I am reminded of her favourite expression. She laughs her hearty laugh that seems to contain her smile, too. "Now I remember why I didn't work in the hospital for long."

Jackie is now eating gluten-free so we order pad Thai for the rice noodles.

"Many nurses say that the emotional aspect of nursing causes burnout. Even young nurses worry about this. They always ask me, 'How do you handle your emotions?' They are taught to hold back and detach themselves, but few can do it.

"Because it's not human. I would challenge that. That approach only gives them the message to be afraid of their emotions, but our emotions are what fuel us as nurses. We should encourage nurses and doctors to be more human and give the kind of care to their patients that they'd like their family member to receive." Jackie looks incredulous at the very idea of "burnout," yet it's widely discussed and researched in my profession. She seems to consider burnout a myth, not the truism some nurses fall back on to explain their discontentment with, or disengagement from, patient care.

"I don't believe in burnout. Burnout is not from caring *too* much, it's from not caring *enough*, starting with ourselves – self-care. Everyone needs to do that, but nurses have to take extra-good care of themselves in order to do this work. I would challenge the whole notion of burnout."

I would challenge that. It's a good phrase, especially in the hospital where there are many bugaboos – like "burnout" – and sacred cows – like dreary waiting rooms or bad hospital food – things that have always been done a certain way but don't even make sense any more. Yet, so often, creativity and initiative are stifled in the big corporate entities that hospitals have become.

I would challenge that. I'm going to keep that phrase handy in my tool kit.

"You know what you should see?" Jackie says to me in the parking lot, as we're about to get into our cars. "VON's hospice. You'll love it. It's not far from here."

"It's on my agenda," I tell her. In fact, it's my next stop.

21

CHERRY BLOSSOMS FOR EVERLASTING LIFE

THIS IS A PLACE WHERE PEOPLE COME TO DIE.

That's all I can think about as I drive an hour from pad Thai with Jackie in London to this grand, stately mansion called Sakura House, in Woodstock, Ontario. It's the last stop on this leg of my itinerary, and I'll drive home later this afternoon.

I turn off the highway onto a long circular driveway, park the car, and walk to the front door of the hospice. On one side of this imposing, but elegant, building is a grove of well-groomed topiary trees. At the other side, tucked discreetly toward the back, is a long ramp sloping down from the back entrance, probably for deliveries and where, I presume, the bodies are taken out, transferred to the hearse, then to the funeral parlour.

On the website they say that a hospice is a place to die with dignity, peace, and comfort.

Where I work, *no one is allowed to die* — at least not without a monumental, *apocalyptic* battle. A hospital death is a hidden, whispered, subversive act; it is a sign of our failure to do what we've implicitly promised.

Nurse Manager Helen Vink waits for me in the airy, spacious front foyer.

"This is the place where I give the first hugs," she says, enveloping me in one.

Helen takes me on a tour, first through the library, then to a sitting room with a Persian rug, a grand piano, and comfortable couches. "We held a wedding here, a day before the mother died." Another room is circular with light-yellow walls and more couches and easy chairs. There is a large bay window and other windows all around.

"One young man with cancer liked to spend his last days in here because of these windows," Helen says. "When it snowed, he said he imagined he was inside a snow globe."

We peek in an empty room, all ready for the next person who will die here. There is a sofa bed, recliner, mini fridge, microwave, a TV, and, on the bed, a colourful, handmade quilt. Each room leads to a patio that overlooks the grounds, with ornamental grasses, a memorial flower garden that blooms in the spring, and a fountain with a pond in which gold and black Koi swim under a thin layer of ice and snow.

Helen and the hospice manager, Robin Kish, tell me about the hospice. The house itself, and its Japanese gardens and estate of seven acres, belonged to Toyota Canada, who sold it for two dollars to VON. In three years, there have been three hundred patients and three hundred deaths. Here, family members can come and go as they please, even stay overnight and sleep on the sofa bed or recliners. Pets are allowed, too. In Japanese, *sakura* means cherry blossom, which is a symbol for everlasting life. In the spring there are real flowers, but now, in winter, vases are filled with ceramic or glass ones. Helen explains that the cherry blossom is a reminder of the shifting seasons, the fleeting nature of human existence, and the impermanence of life.

This would be a nice place to live, I think, as strange as that sounds. It's comfortable and tastefully furnished. It feels inviting and cozy. In the spacious country kitchen I smell fresh coffee and muffins baking in the oven.

What does the ICU smell like? Don't ask. Hopefully, you don't know.

People say it's a relief when they come here, but making the decision can be difficult. Helen tells of a woman with terminal cancer who sat outside in a taxi with the meter running for hours. "She couldn't bring herself to enter because she believed the door swings only one way. We assured her the door can swing the other way, too. She needed to know that it wasn't necessarily the last stop. She had family but didn't tell them she was here. She brought all of her possessions here – there wasn't much – and wouldn't talk to any of us. She died in a week, just as she wanted – to slip away quietly."

Helen calls that a "good death" because the woman died on her own terms. I have seen many deaths, but few I'd call "good." In the hospital, death can be complicated. So often we feel what we're really treating is the family's fear of death. Many deaths are fraught with family conflict and heated emotions. I have witnessed some horrific deaths, so many, in fact, that I have been ruined for knowing what a good death looks like. I'm pleased that Helen is willing to describe it to me.

"People who are dying tell us that they want no rushing around, no pain, to have comfort and maximal mental clarity for as long as possible, and, of course, to have their family and friends close by." She points out that there are no ventilators here, or cardiac monitors, or dialysis machines. There are no oxygen saturation probes, no blood work, and no IVs.

I've always considered these things essential. Come to think of it, I don't think I've ever witnessed the death of a person who didn't have an IV. How does one die without *equipment,* I wonder?

"These technologies do not provide comfort or dignity, which is our focus here," Helen reminds me.

"What about urinary catheters?"

"Only for comfort."

"Feeding tubes?"

"Not here. Feeding tubes make no sense in a hospice. The body does not require food as it is shutting down. We may give small amounts of water or food for comfort. It is more symbolic than anything, but may be meaningful to the family."

Helen says they explain to the family what is happening at each step of the process. "The person's irregular breathing, the gurgling, gasping sounds, may be distressing to the family, but they're a normal part of dying. We medicate for pain or discomfort with the goal of maximizing alertness as a patient progresses toward death."

"'Progresses toward death' is what we call 'worsening' or 'declining,'" I say ruefully. "So, no 'circling the drain?' I take it? No 'crumping,' or 'flat-lining'?" I cringe at saying these coarse terms in this refined and dignified context, but it's true, we commonly use them in the hospital.

"We're death-friendly here. We don't say 'gone on,' 'passed,' or 'not with us anymore.'"

Yet even here, not everyone is in a state of acceptance. Helen tells me of a father who was dying and his wife, who wouldn't tell their children. The daughter at university didn't know her father was in a hospice. "'Tell the kids,' he pleaded, 'I want to see them one last time,' but she wouldn't because she didn't believe he was dying. 'You'll see, he'll walk out of here. He'll be your first to recover,' she said. He asked me to call his kids and I did. His wife was furious, but I had no qualms about it because I was fulfilling the patient's wishes. That's what guides me."

In another situation, a mother knew she was dying but her daughter disagreed with her. The hospice team felt the mother was hanging on for her daughter. "She was a skeleton, you could see every bone, and one day her resps dropped down to four or five a minute. The daughter kept shaking her mother to make her breathe. 'You'll make it to Christmas, Mom,' she told her, and believed it, too. Unfortunately, her mother died before Thanksgiving."

I have a sudden ICU flashback, to a brutal, violent death.

"My husband will not die, do you hear me? Death is not an option," the wife screamed at us, as her husband was exsanguinating. Blood was gushing out of his mouth in spurts with each thrust of CPR. "Don't let this happen!" she

yelled at us. "Do something!" But we were already doing everything. Later, as we cleaned and then wrapped his dead body, we lamented, "He went out in a hail of bullets, a 'blaze of glory,'" befitting a man that the wife described as a "fighter to the end, a man who never gives up."

Most patients say their last wish is to go home. Families want to provide that, but I don't think they are always aware of what they're getting into. Do they know how messy and physically gruelling it is to care for someone who is dying? Can they afford around-the-clock nursing care to supplement home care hours and their own labour? Sometimes the plan is to die at home, but at some point they panic and bring the patient to the emergency department. But a hospice seems like the perfect compromise between home and the hospital. Here, a family can help with caregiving if they wish, or just focus on saying goodbye. Sometimes it can be a long and exhausting vigil, but at least in this home-like place, they can rest near their loved one.

"Here, death decides the pace and it's usually gradual, incremental," Helen says. "It's like lights going out in an apartment building, slowly, one by one. That's how our bodies shut down."

It sounds so gentle the way she describes it. I once heard a doctor ask a patient, "Do you want to die this week or next week?" In the ICU, we can manipulate such things – and we do.

Without knowing it, I chose a good day to visit. There's a potluck Christmas lunch for staff and volunteers and I'm invited to join in the deliciously retro meal, a delightful blast from the past – a repast of Swedish meatballs, devilled eggs, a Jell-O-and-marshmallow mould, sliced ham, soft rolls with butter, and gingerbread cake. After lunch, the nurses gather in the front sitting room to ask my impressions of the hospice.

"It's a beautiful place and it must be very satisfying to work here and get to deliver what you promise – comfort and dignity. In the hospital, people are often disappointed in us when we can't deliver what they expected." They nod in recognition because, like most of us, they started out as hospital nurses. "What's it like to work here?" I ask them.

"You wouldn't do this work if you didn't love it," one nurse says. Other responses are called out as they come to mind.

"Most people don't want to hear about what I do for a living. I tell them I'm a Walmart greeter and they leave me alone."

"Giving someone the gift of a beautiful death balances the sadness we may feel."

"Once we got a standing ovation at a funeral from the family of a man who died with us."

"The sadness gets to me at times, but we check in with each other to see how we're coping."

"You don't realize the weight you carry until you leave for awhile and feel it lift."

"Working here has taught me not to sweat the small stuff. It's made me realize that we don't live forever, that our time here is short."

Nursing teaches you that truth, if nothing else.

"We need to give death the respect and celebration we give lavishly to births, birthdays, and anniversaries," Helen says as the others nod in agreement. "As a society, we need to become involved in deciding how, when, and where we want to die. There should be midwives for death as there are for birth. Maybe this generation will do for death what our generation did for birth." Helen is hopefully wistful. "Just as we de-medicalized labour and delivery, made hospitals more sensitive to families, and brought birthing home, we need to bring death home.

"Six weeks after a death, we call to find out how the family is doing and offer any bereavement support we can," Helen continues. "They are invited to a memorial service that is held for each person who dies at Sakura House. It is organized by the volunteers. Some find it difficult to come back, but when they do they are glad they did."

There's a final ritual that is carried out for each person that dies here, and Helen describes it to me. "The nurses perform the final care, give the last bath. Family members participate if they wish. The person is covered with a quilt and taken out in a procession. The staff line up and stand at attention, like an honour guard, as the person is carried out, their face uncovered. This person who came in the front door now goes out the front door. There is no hiding or shame. We give the family a handmade silk cherry blossom that our volunteers make, and say our goodbyes."

If I told anyone I spent the day at a hospice talking about death, I'm sure they'd look at me in concern. *Oh, how sad that must have been.* And I'd say, no, it wasn't. It was joyful.

I wonder if they'd believe me.

22

360 DEGREES

EVEN ON THIS BITTERLY COLD February morning, the grey and black husky, one blue eye, and one green eye – a dog built for winter – is shivering. He huddles into the crook of the arm of a young boy in a hoodie and ripped jeans who's sitting cross-legged on the street corner shaking a paper cup, coins jingling, in my direction.

I'm not some rich lady! This scarf is polyester – a Hermès knock-off. This necklace is drugstore bling.

Nevertheless.

I open my wallet. Thinking of Wayne and feeling guilty for all that I have and for all that he – and this ragamuffin boy sitting on the sidewalk in front of me – do not, I hand him a twenty-dollar bill. He looks astonished, then embarrassed. Perhaps my largesse makes him feel like he's a particularly needy case.

"I can't take that." He thrusts it back at me. "It's way too much."

"Well, I can't break it. Buy something nice for you and your dog."

"Don't worry about us. We have a place to stay." He looks away. Have I offended him?

Here's a good one: "Knock-knock jokes. Do homeless people get them?"

What do you call a home visit to a person who lives on the street?

A homeless visit.

As I walk along the street toward the nurse practitioner (NP) clinic, a woman dismounts from her bicycle to ask me politely for any spare change, explaining, "It's the end of the month."

I seem to have walked straight into skid row. And where is the sign that says, "Word up, folks. Rich city lady has arrived in town!"

Despite my harmless jocularity, I have a soft spot – even an affinity – for homeless people, even more so after meeting Wayne and hearing his story. But my hospital training has toughened me and I know how to steel myself and put up a wall when I need to. "Sorry," I tell her regretfully, "I'm plumb out of cash." I keep walking.

"My husband is on disability," she calls out after me. "He has anxiety and depression."

"Don't we all?"

Yes, we all have stress, but those of us who have a home, a family, an education, a well-paying job, and a lot of nice things have lots of soft, safe places to fall if we need to. Oh, I've been guilty of all the usual unkind thoughts, stood in silent judgement: *Giving money to panhandlers is futile. . . . It only encourages them. . . . It's a drop in the bucket. . . . They'll use it for drink or drugs. . . . Can't they clean themselves up? . . . Why don't they get a job?* And I've done worse: I have pretended not to see and looked away.

Be nice, I remind and reprimand myself. I want to be nice, but in the few minutes it takes me to walk from my car to the VON 360 Degree Nurse Practitioner–Led Clinic, located in the downtown shopping mall of the sleepy town of Peterborough in South Central Ontario, two more people approach me for a handout. I rush along through the mall to get to the clinic.

The mall itself feels like a community centre. It houses the offices of other charities like United Way, Red Cross, and, of course, VON. It's a hub for the downtrodden, the drunk or high, those who do not have anywhere else to get away from the cold, and all those who have fallen on bad times – they all seem to have gravitated here.

My eye is drawn to a tall, skinny girl who looks about sixteen. She has one hand on a baby stroller and the other holds a few quarters as she stands in front of the "Hurricane Simulator" amusement ride, pondering whether to give it a whirl (with her infant in her arms or by herself?). I sigh, thinking about how much wherewithal and maturity is required to care for a baby, raise a child. Does she have what it takes or at least, the supports to help her?

Now, a nurse is not supposed to have biases or prejudices; being "non-judgemental" is practically a job requirement. Our patients – our clients – whose lives are in our trust, are at their most vulnerable. Think of the scary implications if we ever let any of our personal opinions affect our care. However, I know at times they do. I don't think mine ever have – I hope not – but over all of these years that I've been a nurse, I can't say for certain that they haven't.

A confession of a more trivial *faux pas*: I have developed a mild girl crush on Nurse Practitioner Kathryn Roka, the clinical director of the 360 Clinic. We've only talked on the phone, but I have visited her personal website to learn more about her. From what I can tell, she's brilliant and beautiful, fun-loving – and, best of all, she's a nurse-author like me. She's just published her first book, *Aubrey*. It's part one in an action-packed fantasy trilogy featuring a courageous protagonist who is, *surprise*, a nurse practitioner.

In person, Kathryn is pretty and petite – and a dynamo. A mother, a marathon runner, she is also disarmingly modest – despite the fact that she advertises her book wherever she drives. Her Volkswagen Rabbit is shrink-wrapped, bumper to bumper, in the colourful book cover image of *Aubrey*. "I did it to prevent my son from borrowing the car," she says with a hearty belly laugh, surprising from someone so petite and elegant.

We sit in her tiny, cramped office, jam-packed with stacks of books and journals. (No paper patient charts here; all the medical records are electronic.) The walls are crowded with family photographs and a hand-painted sign that says, "People who say it can't be done should not interrupt those who are doing it." Kathryn has given me a tour of this immaculate, modern clinic, and now we take a few minutes to chat before her first client arrives. To be honest, I don't really know what an NP does, so Kathryn explains.

"Prevention, teaching, and counselling. We work independently and can diagnose, prescribe, treat, make a referral, admit or discharge to a hospital."

"It sounds like what a general practitioner does."

"Yes, it is," she says with her confident smile. "We share the same knowledge base and skill set, but we work differently. For what ails most people, a nurse practitioner is the right person. If you need open-heart surgery – that's something else. You'll understand more after today," she promises. "Any more questions? Fire away."

"Do you treat people of all ages?"

"Yup, from womb to tomb. We have a pediatric suite with an examining table that is a smiling turquoise dinosaur named Monty. We also treat teenagers, many 'at-risk youth,' who are dealing with addictions, poverty, homelessness, mental illness, and gender confusion."

I wonder if the boy with the dog on the street corner knows about this place.

"Babies, too?"

"Yes. In fact, our first client was a baby. She was left on the doorstep on the day the clinic opened. The mother was never located but the father came forward to claim the baby. With lots of support, he is now raising her on his own."

Kathryn has a down-home style, a beautiful smile that appears readily, and intelligent, twinkling eyes. She's glamorous, too, dressed in black pants and a black-and-white blouse. (Black-and-white is her signature look.) She explains that she runs the clinic in a "nurse practitioner" way, always ensuring that ample time is booked for each patient so as to allow conversations to unfold and flow at their own pace.

"We never want to hurry people along. We're not managers or business people, so we have a lot to learn, but we know what we want and I've set the bar high."

They offer extended hours and off-hours services. Same-day access is important, so the office manager and receptionists always carve out time for walk-ins. This clinic is funded by the government and also by private businesses and philanthropic donations. As word is getting around town, the practice here is growing quickly. Kathryn has hired two NPs, with plans to hire more, two social workers, a dietician, and a pharmacist and two nurses. "At times, we are running on fumes, but we never turn anyone away. What helps make us so efficient is that our two RNs practise to their full scope."

"Full-scope" practice is a hot-button issue. It boils down to the fact that nurses have been underutilized. We have a lot more skills than we think we do. For whatever reason, nurses have held ourselves back from working to the full scope of our practice.

I ask Kathryn to put it into terms I can picture.

"The RNs in this clinic do full physical exams." She uses the fingers of both hands to list their other capabilities: "Pap smears, pelvic exams, cancer screening, well-baby visits, triage acute patients, counselling, health teaching, chronic disease management. Soon, RNs will be able to dispense and even prescribe certain medications. Our two RNs, Katy and Elena, will tell you more about that. The point is, they do everything that they have the skill, knowledge, and judgement to do. It expands what we can offer our clients."

This clinic cares for people who have complex, often chronic, problems. Many have never used the health care system before and have "complicated lives," as Kathryn puts it. They are dealing with poverty, addictions, mental health issues. "Primary care is a different way of thinking about health. It looks at everything – medication, diet, lifestyle to help improve health and prevent disease. We spend a lot of time with each person and we're in it for the long haul, not just when they have a problem."

The clients she will see today have all agreed to have me sit in on their appointments.

The first one, Oliver, walks in with a professorial manner. He's a portly but distinguished-looking man in his mid-fifties, wearing a tweed blazer, carrying a thin briefcase, with an unlit pipe in his mouth and a cell phone wrapped in bits of torn newspaper and hanging from his neck by a piece of binder twine. Oliver is delighted to see Kathryn and to meet me. He even shakes my hand with a slight ceremonial bow.

Kathryn hones right in on her first concern. She tells Oliver that the lab found trace amounts of blood in his stool. She has ruled out active bleeding since his hemoglobin is normal and unchanged, and it could be a "false positive" for cancer, but to be sure, she wants him to have a colonoscopy. He recoils at her suggestion and folds his arms in protest. Over the top of her computer, level with his eyes, she looks at him squarely, unequivocally. "This test will offer you a huge reassurance or it will save your life."

Kathryn turns to me. "I have caught many colon cancers. It's always best to find pathologies as early as possible."

To help Oliver warm up to the idea, she offers a tip for the unpleasant preparation. "Choose the salty solution, not the sweet one. First, freeze your mouth with an ice cube. Have a glass of water ready. Throw the stuff back like a shooter, then down the water."

They've been chatting casually for a few minutes, so when she gets up to take his blood pressure, there's no chance of white-coat hypertension. "But," she says, "if you've had even one cigarette in the previous hour, it will give a false elevation."

"You know I quit smoking, Kathryn," he says with a coy, unconvincing look.

But he walked in with a pipe in his mouth! Didn't she notice that?

Oliver's pressure continues to be high, and since it has been resistant to dietary changes, weight loss, and the medications she's prescribed, Kathryn has decided to send him to a cardiologist, but she cautions him, "I've told you, Oliver. This cardiologist is very good, but he will only address your heart issues. Don't expect more than that."

"Thanks, I need the warning."

Together they review his health risks. By using a chart, they discover that with Oliver's medical profile, the odds of him having a cardiac event are very high. Oliver's father died from heart disease, so
heredity is also a factor.

Kathryn discloses something personal. "I'll tell you both a secret.
The reason that my passion for heart health is particularly *heart-felt* is
that my father died from a cardiac arrest at the age of forty-seven." I'm
impressed by her willingness to be so frank and vulnerable.

"Heart health. We always talk about that, don't we, Oliver? I'm on
it. I want to bring your LDL down. A moderate amount of alcohol helps
lower cholesterol, but I don't want you to take this recommendation
too far. Alcohol's an issue, too, isn't it?" She gives him a playful wink.
"But one thing at a time."

He looks overwhelmed and admits, "I am having trouble coming to
terms with it all. But I am lucky. When I had a doctor, he'd only discuss
one problem at a time. If there was a second problem I had to book
another appointment. 'No ticky, no washy.' Kathryn has a job to do and
so do I – to be a responsible patient and do what we decide I need to do.
But" – he folds his hands and sits up straight – "I will not take the iron
pills you've prescribed."

"That's fine, Oliver. I support that. We'll do a complete review of
your meds at our next visit."

"Such a rigamarole." He gives a resigned sigh. "I am coming to the
realization I am not immortal. I am a gentleman with diabetes, lung
problems, high blood pressure. But the iron pills are terrible. They
gave me constipation. Very unpleasant. I will not take them."

"I support that," Kathryn repeats and moves on to bowel habits.
"We live in a constipated society. Here's what I do. Every morning, I
sit on the toilet, whether I feel I have to go or not. This is how you
train yourself to have a natural bowel movement first thing in the
morning." She turns to Oliver. "What are you doing about exercise?"

"I walk the cat." He grins at her and Kathryn erupts in her unexpectedly boisterous laugh.

"Kathryn's put me through the car wash." Though he tries to act disgruntled, he's anything but. "This is the best medical care I've ever received." He shows us a graph he's been keeping on his own of the past two months of daily blood pressure recordings and points to a row of peaks. "Here, I ran out of my beta blocker."

"I'll make sure to give you a refill this time," Kathryn promises.

Together Kathryn and Oliver look at a recent chest x-ray and review the results of his pulmonary function tests. Kathryn is waiting for a report from the nephrologist she sent him to because of his mildly elevated glomerular filtration rate, an early sign of kidney failure.

I'm beginning to connect the dots. Many of our critically ill patients in the ICU have one or more, or all, of these conditions, making their survival rates poor. What if you could get at them "before," in the early stages of their disease, rather than "after," when we treat them in the ICU and they are often at the end-stage of their health problems? Suddenly, the prospect of working on this side seems appealing, even exciting.

In between clients, Kathryn explains more. "When Oliver first came, I noticed precancerous lesions on his tongue. We got him to stop smoking."

"But he walked in with a pipe," I point out.

"It's a prop!" And again, I get to hear that great big laugh explode from her, her body so compact and her demeanour so composed.

Kathryn tells me how she became an NP. She used to be a law clerk on Bay Street, doing sexy deals and living a glamorous life. At the age of thirty-five, she became terribly ill. "I had a raging fever and went into liver failure. My stool turned white, my urine was black as Coca-Cola. It was acute mononucleosis. When I recovered, I decided to become a nurse, but when I graduated I knew the hospital wasn't for me. I need *sleep*."

Kathryn worked in public health at a computer job, but one long weekend in May at a pool party, a friend suggested she'd make a good nurse practitioner. "I had no idea what it involved, but I called. Unbelievably, on a long-weekend Monday, someone answered." Kathryn makes a telephone of her fingers and talks into her palm, the receiver. "They'd just had a cancellation, so there was a spot for me. 'I think I'm in,' I said to my friends. It was meant to be. Call it divine intervention."

As we wait for her next client Kathryn explains that "360" is not just the street number. It's meant to indicate that this is a full-service facility. She likes the message it sends about turning people's lives around. Most of all, it pays homage to our Aboriginal population, to whom the circle symbolizes returning home, wholeness. The chief of a local tribe performed a smudge ceremony at the clinic's opening ceremony.

Kathryn introduces her next patient. "Meet Meg, our poster child for the 360."

It's hard to believe Meg was once a heroin addict. She looks robustly healthy, radiantly happy. I would have guessed Meg is around fifty, but not so. "I'm pushing sixty-five," she reveals. "When I was using, I looked eighty. Now, I get enough sleep. I take vitamins. I come here. I'm dealing with my problems."

"We got you off cigarettes, didn't we?" Kathryn prompts.

Meg nods. "I want to be here for my grandchildren. I've cut out alcohol, improved my diet."

"What about exercise? Can we do anything about that?" Kathryn asks. "Your blood pressure is still high at 178 over 90 today." She decides to increase the dose of Meg's anti-hypertension medication and explains the importance of one of her other medications. "Statins. They're our best weapon against cholesterol buildup. No one is going to have elevated cholesterol on my watch."

Meg looks over at Kathryn affectionately. "I trust her. She's changed my life, just knowing she's in my corner."

"Trust. It's the only way to develop a partnership." Kathryn smiles at Meg.

Her story of recovery is inspiring.

"When I was using, I lied, stole, cheated, conned. I worked the streets for drugs and I needed the drugs to work the streets. I thought I'd never be able to crawl out of that hell. Somehow I got to this clinic and met Kathryn. She gave me the message, *I believe in you. You can beat this thing and I will help you in any way I can.* When someone like her says that to you, you feel maybe there's a chance. I came from Vancouver's Eastside, the worst drug haven in the country. Now, I have a future, the respect of my family. I can hold my head up. I don't go to support sessions because people there have a 'poor me' mentality. I don't want to hear garbage talk. It's not how long you've been abstinent, but the quality of your sobriety. I'd rather be with someone who's been clean a few months but has a good attitude than someone who's been clean a few years and gripes all the time."

Meg still takes methadone, to keep her off heroin. She's happy to teach me about the drug, as I know nothing about it. "It's a synthetic heroin. It's mixed in orange juice in a controlled dose so you can't overdose. That way, your veins don't get wrecked and you don't get hepatitis. If you're not clean you have to come into the clinic to get it every day and that's a horrible place. After awhile, I got 'carries' to take home, which was more convenient for me."

Meg had been using heroin to obliterate the memory of a childhood trauma.

"But I can't tell you about it." She closes her eyes for a moment. "It still affects me. I ache inside. Bad stuff happened. The other day, I saw some one on the street scrounging for butts. Not long ago, that was me. I was the one going through garbage cans looking for something to eat or smoke."

Sometimes, there really are happy endings.

After Meg, Sean strides in with confidence, in a black leather jacket and tight jeans. He's a bit rough around the edges, but handsome in a tough, rugged sort of way. He has a shoulder injury, but seems to forget about that when he gets to what he really came to tell me.

"When I used to have a problem, I'd go to the ED. I only came to this clinic to get a prescription refill, but she" – he points at Kathryn, pre- tending to accuse her – "wanted to do more. I want my wife to come, too, but she says she'll only go to a doctor. 'Why?' I ask. I get everything I need here. What I like about this place is that they're not bossy. I don't like anyone telling me what to do. But I have stopped buying my smokes from the reserve, even though they're cheaper, because Kathryn told me they're full of poison."

"Many of the toxins in cigarettes are the same as the ones in lawn pesticides, rat poison, lighter fluid, and rocket fuel, and yet we voluntarily inhale them into our precious bodies?" Kathryn asks. "Sean, you tell me when you want to stop smoking altogether. We'll be waiting to help you when you're ready."

"I'll let you know."

"I'll support you wherever you're at with it." She turns to a new subject. "Okay, how about sex? How long's it been?"

Sean has erectile dysfunction, and Kathryn has told him that can be an early sign of heart disease. The arteries in the penis are the smallest in the body so they're the first to clog up, preventing an erection. Smoking and alcohol can decrease function, too. Kathryn hands him a pack of drug samples. "Try these and enjoy. If your erection lasts for more than three hours, go to the emergency department."

"Just like they say on TV. So, what do they do for that? Send me to the head nurse?"

Kathryn turns to me. "I always talk to my clients about sex. They usually don't raise the topic themselves but it's an important human need. Elders especially crave touch, being hugged. For some patients, I actually prescribe sex."

"What's the recommended dosage?" I joke. She laughs with me, but she's serious about the therapeutic benefits of sexual health, listing its cardio benefits, endorphin production, and depression-boosting effects related to right prefrontal cortex stimulation.

She returns to Sean. "Is there anything else I can help you with today?"

"How to survive without hockey." He looks glum. There's been an NHL strike and there's no sign of resolution.

"Sorry, can't help you with that," she says cheerfully, obviously not a hockey fan.

"Well, I still have shoulder pain but I go to physio and try to keep a stiff upper lip," he says, then mutters under his breath, "Let's hope something gets stiff."

Kathryn moves on. "How about booze?"

"Not much. I've cut back. I drink it for the buzz, not the taste."

"What about a change to light beer? Make an agreement with yourself, not me."

"The treatment I get here is excellent," Sean tells me as he stands up to leave. "I feel the people here are genuinely concerned for my well-being. There's no bullshit. From day one I had trust in this place. I'm never rushed and I never have to wait. Honestly, I think Kathryn cares more about me than I do. They gotta clone her."

As we wait for the next client, Kathyn notes, "We often have late arrivals or no-shows. Not everyone can organize life like we do." She points at our smartphones and daily organizers.

Jade walks in tentatively. She is thin with a sallow complexion and looks frail, but summons impressive vehemence to express her anger at Kathryn.

"Why didn't you refill my pain meds? When they weren't with my other meds, I had a panic attack. My body was vibrating. It put me in a dark place. How could you do this to me?" Her fists are clenched at her sides and her eyes are blazing with rage.

"The medication you are asking for is not the norm for what you describe as depression and fibromyalgia."

"You made my condition worse because you wouldn't order my pain meds. I had to go to two doctors to get what I need. I didn't want to get into such a bad state that I'd end up having to go to the hospital."

Kathryn sits calmly. "I'm sorry I can't give you what you want —"

"But there are *doctors* out there who will. Why won't you?"

"Oxycodone is not the drug you need, and it has side effects, as you know. These may not be the answers that you want to hear, but —"

"But some doctors do have the answers! I've tried the antidepressants, pain patches. Nothing works except the oxys. I can't seem to get across to you the urgency of my situation."

"It's not in your best interest to order that medication," Kathryn says kindly but firmly.

"I'm on only six, sometimes eight, per day. I'd love to be off altogether, but I have pain. You don't believe me."

"I do believe you and I want you to keep coming here."

"I'll only come if you'll help me."

"I want to help you. You are important to this practice."

Tears spring to Jade's eyes as her anger breaks. "The thing is, I think you actually mean it."

"I do, but I don't want this clinic to be known as an easy place to get narcotics."

Looking both vindicated and victimized, Jade appeals to me. "I've tried to educate Kathryn about fibromyalgia. That it's an individual thing. That it's caused by emotional trauma. There's one drug that gives me relief, but she" – Jade stops to flash a scornful look at Kathryn, who is unperturbed – "won't order it for me. She only knows what the textbook says." Jade glowers at her. "Educate yourself," she scolds. "Use your brain." She jabs at the side of her head. "Why did you do that to me?" She starts to cry.

Kathryn hands her a box of tissues. "As I told you, Jade, I can't substantiate ordering that drug for this diagnosis."

"Lots of people in my fibromyalgia support group get this drug from their doctor. Why won't you order it for me? At first, when you didn't renew my pain meds, I was scared. Now, I'm angry." Her face is tight and twisted. "I don't want to end up in hospital. They treat you like shit in there. I'd rather die than go to the hospital." Jade storms out of Kathryn's office in a huff, her problem far from resolved. Kathryn turns away from her computer, crosses her legs, and swivels her chair to face me. "So, what do you think? What's your impression?" she asks me.

"Typical drug-seeking behaviour. Jade tried to manipulate you, but you didn't budge. Why didn't you tell her she's addicted and recommend she go to rehab?"

"She's not ready to hear that and I haven't won her trust. Not yet, anyway. I hope to in time."

We turn to other matters as we wait for the next patient.

I ask Kathryn about the turf wars I've heard about between doctors and NPs.

"In my experience, you get treated the way you act. Our focus is prevention, theirs is treatment. It's different. We do not replace doctors, but we can diagnose, prescribe, order tests — everything a general practitioner does. It sounds radical but back in the sixties RNs weren't even allowed to take blood pressure — that was something only a doctor could do."

"Do doctors see NPs as competition, taking patients away?"

"Most see the relationship as collaboration. We don't make as much money as they do and we cost the health care system a lot less, but there's more than enough work for all of us. We need to play nicely together in the sandbox. It's best for patient care."

"I have heard them express concerns about safety. They say, how can a nurse with two extra years of education equal eight years of medical school?"

"It's a reasonable question," Kathryn admits, but doesn't know the answer. "Even skeptical doctors admit they haven't had safety concerns so far, but time will tell." She thinks it over and has something more to say. "Concerns about safety? Here's what's not safe. Recently, I had a patient with right lower quadrant pain and all five signs of acute appendicitis, including McBurney's. I prepared a note, sent her to the ER and I called them, too, to tell them she was coming. She ended up sitting for ten hours in the ER because, as they told me later, 'We don't read NP's notes. We make our own diagnoses.' Of course, it ruptured. I was livid. Yes, there are still pockets of resistance, but overall I'd say it's improving."

Kathryn sees more clients — Sebastian, a morbidly obese man with sickle cell anemia who suffers from depression and poverty. He's a lovely, sensitive gentleman, soft-spoken and truly sad. After tweaking his meds and renewing his prescriptions, Kathryn takes time to look at the cartoons he's brought to show her. He is creating a graphic novel about death as opposed to attempting suicide himself. Kathryn treats a woman for her migraines, then a teenager with an infected ear piercing with whom she also manages to do some counselling about safe sex. By the afternoon, Kathryn is still going strong, but I need a break.

"What's the most important thing I can help you with today?" I hear her say to the next client and as I duck out of her examining room to take a break and stretch my legs, I run into Krystina Nickerson, one of the 360 social workers. She looks *waaay* cool and badass in jeans and a denim jacket, sporting an asymmetrical haircut with blue highlights, a peacock feather tat on her left foot, and a dancing cherub behind her ear. She invites me into her small, cozy lair of an office, to tell me about her role in this clinic.

"How does the word get out that this town is the place to come if you've hit hard times?"

Peterborough was a once thriving town, Krystina explains. Geographically, it's at the crossroads of small town and big city, and the gateway to the northern, more rural areas of the province of Ontario. Like many small towns these days, the middle-class jobs are gone. Canada Packers, General Electric, Quaker Oats, and Westclox are all successful companies that closed their offices here because of the free-trade agreement with the U.S. and the downturn in the economy. All that's left are dollar stores, cheap shoe outlets, and little emporiums that sell beach towels, cheap luggage, and velvet paintings. This town has developed the services that the down-and-out need.

"We have soup kitchens, food banks, drop-in centres, and shelter beds, but without affordable housing, without work, people feel shame. Most want to get off welfare, but they've become demoralized, depressed, and desperately poor. Some are suicidal and turn to alcohol and drugs. Many have fallen victim to addictions. It's a harsh world and they are some of our most vulnerable. They need our protection."

Krystina practises "narrative therapy," which asks, "What is the person's story?" and examines the meaning of life events to that indi-vidual. She connects her clients to political activist groups, like the Rainbow Coalition, LGBTQ youth groups, and sex-worker's rights' groups. "Being involved politically gives people a sense of control over oppressive forces."

She works from a "non-oppressive world view," and is critical of the failed strategies of law enforcement and prohibition, as well as abstinence requirements and punishing systems. Krystina believes that a solution is to embrace a harm reduction approach that would include safe-injection sites, methadone clinics, and needle exchange.

"Where did you learn this grassroots, radical style? At home, from your parents?"

She laughs at that idea. "They learned from me!"

Her hard-core, liberal, political stance is so completely at odds with my more traditional, conservative hospital sensibility that it takes me aback. But I can feel myself opening to this way of thinking, especially when Krystina confirms the prejudice that Jade reported she'd experi-enced in the hospital. I hate to think that happens, but I know that it does. I wish I could say that we weren't that way, but there are still hos-pital staff who see the word "addict'" or "IV drug user" or "homeless" in the patient's chart and label and stigmatize that person. When patients come into the ICU "with no fixed address," with lice or scabies or track marks or nicotine-stained fingers, we rush to clean them up, scrub them down, disinfect them, and feel we've done our duty. But our actions speak volumes; I am mortified to realize how unsuccessful many of us are at stamping out our biases, or at least at keeping our judgments silent and invisible.

The phone rings and Krystina takes the call. I eavesdrop on her conversation. "Cool. I'm glad you're okay . . . I want you to get your butt back in here . . . you're going through a rough time . . . I want to hear all about it."

Her softly lit office has a bookshelf filled with gifts from clients. On the wall is a framed sign that says, "You may not be bigoted . . . but that comment was." On a corner table there are smooth stones, each with painted messages: "No Means No"; "Consent is Sexy." Many of Krystina's clients are sex-trade workers whose erratic, chaotic lifestyles make it hard to keep appointments, so once a week, the clinic hosts a drop-in potluck with an NP, an RN, and a social worker on duty. They also offer access to a shower, toiletries, clean clothes, washer and dryer.

Krystina gets off the phone and we turn to the subject of safe-injection sites, but my hospital way of thinking gets in my way again. "Harm reduction" strategies are a hard sell, especially to those of us who work in the hospital.

"Doesn't that merely encourage the addictive behaviour, by making it easier, more readily available? Don't you feel it's *enabling* them?"

"No one – and I mean *no one* – would be on these substances if they didn't have to be. They all want to get off. Harm reduction recognizes this reality and keeps people safer by reducing infections and over-doses, rather than requiring abstinence, which is too demanding for most people." She offers me a rudimentary example of harm reduc-tion thinking.

"Take handouts to panhandlers. People say they'll only spend it on booze or drugs. A harm reduction approach argues that, yes, they use these substances, but at least you reduce the likelihood they'll obtain them in dangerous or illegal ways."

Krystina makes a convincing argument, but I cannot imagine myself giving out crack mouthpieces, clean needles, and syringes to heroin addicts. I can't see myself working in a safe-injection site, advising people how not to overdose, helping someone find a useable vein to shoot – though these are things that street nurses commonly do.

"You could once you realize that drug addiction is a life-threatening condition. You'll have a better appreciation for harm reduction once you realize that this approach saves lives. All harm reduction is," Krystina says, "is about not judging or giving advice."

"What I do realize is that in order to be that way, you need to know the person's story."

She nods. "Their story tells you who they are, it takes you to where they are."

And where I am right now is finished — at least for today.

Kathryn has invited me out to dinner and we're ravenous. We put on our coats, scarves, gloves, and boots to walk to the Indian restaurant around the corner. The thought of samosas, a fiery vindaloo curry, a vegetable biryani with a Kingfisher beer is making my mouth water. But just as we're about to go out the front entrance, a young girl, hugely pregnant, arrives at the door, a tall, skinny guy trailing right behind her. Both wear flimsy jackets and look around seventeen or eighteen. Are they trying to escape the cold or are they looking for narcotics? My guard shoots up. Are there any controlled drugs on the premises? Kathryn and I are here alone. It's already dark. Reaching into my coat pocket for my keys and phone, I plan our getaway.

"I'm hungry." The girl giggles. The boy tries to grope her but she shoves him away.

Kathryn goes to the kitchen where she finds a box of crackers, some packages of pudding, milk, and a bottle of vitamins.

"Serena stopped coming for prenatal care — that's always a huge red flag to alert us to put in a call to Children's Aid, which, by law, I had to do," she tells me. "One day she brought in a urine sample to prove she's clean so she can keep her baby, but I had to dump it. It's worthless if I haven't seen her produce it. She's still using so we told her we'd have to apprehend her baby as soon as it's born until she's well enough to look after it herself."

"How did she take that?"

"Not well. She was furious. She left the clinic, laughing her head off, calling out to us, 'Try to catch me if you can.' I asked the Children's Aid worker, 'How do you do this work? How do you sleep at night?' 'By knowing I am keeping babies safe,' she said."

As we go back out to give Serena the food, Kathryn lowers her voice. "At first, we supported their relationship, until we discovered it was abusive. He's pleasant tonight, but he has a violent side. She needs to step up and make better choices. If she's not able to do that, we'll have to step in."

Serena takes the few supplies gratefully. She tries to brush away the boyfriend, who is swooping at her again. She tries to act annoyed. "Remember what happened last time?" I wonder if "last time" refers to the bruises on her face and neck or her pregnancy? He tugs at her skimpy jacket, trying to cover it over her belly. Then they sail out into the cold, dark night, arms entwined, chirping back and forth to one another like love birds.

Catch me if you can.

I radio a message to the new life on the way. *Stay where you are, as long as you can. It's safe in there, and warm, too. Out here might not be.*

Kathryn and I look at each other. I turn off the lights and she locks the door behind us.

After an encounter as unsettling as that, most people would think it impossible – even unconscionable – to enjoy a nice meal over carefree conversation, yet that's exactly what we do. I know. I know. It seems so unfeeling – even callous – but Kathryn and I are seasoned nurses. Serena is not the first, nor the last. We can't fix everything, but we are dedicated to spending our days making a start. So, yes, we enjoy the dinner and each other's company, and, at the same time, we hold the girl, the boy, and the baby on its way in our minds, in our hearts.

23

BEYOND ALL PREJUDICE

WHEN KATHRYN MENTIONED that the RNs in the clinic work to the "full scope," I was intrigued to know more. This term is often bandied about, but what does it actually look like in the real world? Nurses tend to underestimate, not overestimate, their capacity to take action. It's a timidity born from years of feeling subservient to doctors and a long history of reactive behaviour, rather than taking initiative. So, I'm interested to sit down with the RNs of the 360 Clinic to learn more about their role. Elena is slim and graceful, with salt-and-pepper hair. A few years younger than me, her two kids are still school-aged. Katy has long blond hair in a swingy ponytail and is eight months pregnant. She'll soon be off on a year-long maternity leave.

The conversation starts and flows along with little prompting from me.

KATY: Helping people who are struggling with life is rewarding. It's more real than nursing in the regimented hospital environment and there's more opportunity to be creative. Besides, people don't live their lives on a hospital schedule, by our rules — *you can't sleep in, you have to take your pills when we say* — and it's so noisy, even at night. And yes, it can be challenging to do a dressing change in someone's filthy home where flies are buzzing around or a cat is walking over your sterile field, but you have to show respect and improvise on the spot.

ME: Do you have areas of specialty?

KATY: I love wounds! The drippiest, most infected, complicated, and challenging wounds are my favourites. Said like a true nurse, right? It's tangible evidence that what you're doing is really helping. I've done some extra courses on wound care, since it's my forte. We have a surprising number of clients here with wounds. We have some very *sick* people here.

ME: You say "sick" like we do in the ICU, about patients we're particularly worried about.

KATY: That's true out here, too. My other specialty area is foot care, counselling about pain control and diabetic management, plus I run support groups for tobacco cessation.

ELENA: My particular interest is mental health, especially people living with depression. My other areas of focus are COPD and hypertension. These are some of the clients I'm working with right now.

ME: It seems to me that to care for this population, you have to get over your own prejudices and biases, if you happen to have any.

KATY: I've always worked with this population and have enjoyed it. I do have a problem with infestations. I'm not big on them. Don't get me wrong. I'll deal with it, but I have a phobia.

ELENA: Sometimes it's hard for me with pregnant moms who don't take care of themselves or their kids. This morning, my appointment with a sixteen-year-old girl and her baby was a no-show. When I think of all that it takes to be a parent – and she can't even make it to her child's appointments for a checkup? It's disheartening. But it absolutely breaks my heart when I see neglect, especially of children. I take my role as a mom so seriously. There's a woman I'm working with now. She's a twenty-five-year-old sex-trade worker who came in wearing a mini-skirt in the middle of winter. She's a drug user, using bad heroin with baking soda mixed in, and had huge, inflamed abscesses along the veins on both arms. Every night she bounces from couch to couch. Then she tells me she's pregnant. It's hard to sit by and watch her make choices that are affecting another life.

KATY: I am prepared to deal with the reality of what's out there. It's not always pretty and it's not what I want for myself or my child, but it's easy for me to say that. I've had a different upbringing. Sometimes you struggle to understand people's choices. I took care of one woman who had a huge, infected wound on her vulva. "Will you let me put a dressing on it?" I asked her. "It will get in the way of my work," she said. "An open, infected wound will get also get in the way of your work," I told her and tried to reason with her, but in the end, I could only give her a bunch of supplies, show her how to clean it, and away she went. I haven't seen her since. She had just taken a hit and was high, so I don't know how much sunk in.

ELENA: One of my clients had been in hospital for septicemia and IV antibiotics. Only forty years old, they made her a DNR so there would be no resuscitation in the event of an arrest. They went ahead and made that decision based on their *impression* of her, without even discussing it with her. Another patient had severe anxiety and was suicidal. She also had pneumonia, but that was overlooked. The mental health issue becomes the sole focus – or the opposite happens, where the focus is the medical problems and their mental or emotional state is ignored. These complex patients have the highest needs, but often get the worst care. When we send them to the hospital and they get treated like that, we destroy the trust we've worked so hard to build. We once had a patient in respiratory distress, but he refused to go to the hospital because of the way he was treated the last time. Already in the emergency department, they feel the disgust that people there have for them.

ME: What's it like working with nurse practitioners?

KATY: I haven't worked with doctors. The hospital never appealed to me. I can't imagine having to hunt down a doctor when I need one, or the rudeness that my friends who work in hospitals deal with. Here, it's not like that. There's no hierarchy. Also, there isn't the tension that comes from billing for services. We're all on salary here and spend as much time as each patient needs. Here, the philosophy is holistic nursing, looking at the physical, social, mental, spiritual – all with a focus on prevention. Here, we all speak the same language.

ELENA: Yes, there is no conflict of interest that you have with piecework or private health care. There's no profit motive. It's just about what the patient needs. Sometimes I think about becoming an NP myself, but I know I'd miss being an RN. Being able to diagnose and prescribe is not really my thing. I like the conversations, the picking up the pieces, the coordination of it all.

KATY: Yeah, I like sneaky assessments, like looking like you're doing one thing but at the same time doing another. Having a conversation, but really figuring out what the client needs and how you can help. I'm not the authoritative figure. I leave that to the NPs. For example, when I do tobacco-cessation groups, I tell them about my own experience with smoking and how I struggled with quitting for many years. The main thing is to keep them coming back.

ELENA: We hope that any patient who's fallen off the wagon or has had a setback of any kind feels comfortable coming back here. They know we won't scold them or make them feel guilty. We never give up on anyone. I tell them, I don't care what you do; you'll never get fired from this clinic, even if you relapse.

KATY: Relapse is good, I tell them. Then we can look at it and figure it out. Now you know. It's good that you came back. If you relapse, that's fine. Just keep coming back.

ELENA: The main message is that we're here for you if you want to stop or cut back.

ME: What's your work schedule like?

KATY: Tuesdays and Wednesdays, I'm the go-to RN and Elena has her booked appointments for counselling and diabetic teaching. The

other days we switch. We each have programs we are responsible
for, like COPD, hepatitis, prenatal care, and sexual health.

ELENA: We have same-day spots because there are always some walk-in
clients, so we make sure to be flexible. So many people only want a
quick fix, like at a walk-in clinic. But here, we're like, "Let's talk."
They have to put in the work. It takes time.

KATY: That reminds me of a client I am working with now. He is overweight, diabetic, and inactive, but wants me to help him apply for
a scooter. Meanwhile, he's still walking around. "That's the only
exercise you get," I told him. "If you get the scooter, you won't even
be doing that." Actually, we had a laugh over that together.

ELENA: People test you all the time. One patient was on 110 mg of methadone a day, which is a huge amount. Yet, she was exhibiting
aggressive behaviour. We had a conversation and she admitted she
had a stash of carries. We try to build trust so they can be honest
with us. Some of our clients come to us because they've been "fired"
by their family doctor. That would never happen here. These are
people whose lives are not straight and reliable. Many people have
chaotic lives. If you can't afford food, or if you're in a rooming
house or shelter, if you're depressed or have no transportation, it's
understandable that you might miss an appointment. Home is the
place where you take care of yourself. How can you be healthy if you
don't have a roof over your head? It's basic. If we can't get them in
here, we know we'll see them when they get their welfare cheques
and can buy a bus ticket. We see them if we hold a potluck lunch. We
choose a date just before they get their welfare cheque because
that's when they need it the most.

KATY: Our clinic is not going to save society, but on an individual basis,
one by one, we can make huge improvements in people's lives. We
had a client who was in his mid-fifties, living in a rural area, with zero
money. Mentally, he was very disturbed with paranoia, aggression,
and hallucinations. He also had diabetes. He was so lost, so alone. He
missed too many appointments with his psychiatrist, so she dropped

him. We arranged for him to see a psychiatrist in our telemedicine
network by video-conferencing. The psychiatrist was in Toronto and
the patient was here. We found him housing. "You guys helped me,
my mind is clear." Now, he has a job with a trucking company. Another
guy walked around with only socks on his feet all winter. He had
swelling in his legs, infections, and urinary and bowel incontinence
that led to behaviour issues where he'd throw his stool all over the
room in the shelter. The psychiatrist said he was a medical patient,
the doctors said he was a psych patient. Meanwhile, he was so lonely,
tortured by nightmares, and kept being bounced around from place
to place. He'd go to the emergency department two or three times a
day out of sheer loneliness. When they discovered he had a year-old
untreated hip fracture, that got him admitted to the hospital. We went
there, showered him, took care of the wounds on his feet and his
infections. I can't say all's well with him but he's definitely doing
better. Families sometimes give up on these people. That's so sad.

ELENA: There was another lady, very low-functioning, barely thriving,
malnourished, with poor hygiene, and rotting teeth. We brought
her here and got her blood pressure under control. We did her
laundry, then showed her how to do it herself. With her, we had to
work hard to build up trust. Eventually, we got her shelter in a local
motel, even though she was a smoker. But we saw a huge turn-
around with her, even in that gross motel that was overrun with
mice. She had socks, a bed, a TV. We brought her food. It was more
than she'd ever had, so she was happy. She's in long-term care now
and very content. Many people are isolated like that. There are literally thousands of people in this country who have absolutely no
one to care for them.

KATY: The survival of the human spirit – we see a lot of that here. So
many of our clients have been kicked down, have no hope – it's
inspiring to see them make even small steps.

ELENA: It's sad, but we also see so many inspirational stories of courage. We cope by working together closely and supporting one

another. This work is very rewarding. To me, it is very meaningful. You are accompanying people on their journey. That's why I love this population. They are literally on the margins of society. Primary care is all about building relationships.

KATY: As nurses, you cannot be detached. In school, they teach you to keep a distance, that it's not healthy to get emotionally involved. It's never been that way for me. I feel a lot of emotions for the people who come to this clinic and I like feeling those emotions, whatever they are. I don't shy away from feelings. It's life. It's real. It's their life and you're sharing it with them. Why wouldn't I feel for them?

Another NP in the clinic is Donna Dailey who almost didn't become a nurse, much less a nurse practitioner. "I finished high school at sixteen and you had to be seventeen to apply to nursing school. I was too impatient to wait, so I became a paralegal." She's a full-figured gal after my own heart, stylish with brilliant white hair, black jeans, a tomato-red blazer, and funky red boots. It took twenty-two more years for Donna to find her way to nursing. At first she worked in a GP's office as a family practice nurse doing well-baby exams, vitals, immunizations, and reviewing lab results. Nine years later, when her kids were grown up and she was a grandmother, Donna studied to become an NP, but her husband was in a terrible car accident and she became his caregiver. Her father became terminally ill and was dying as she wrote her final exam.

"As soon as I was done, I flew home to be with him. When I received my diploma and licence in the mail, I didn't even care. It didn't feel worth all the work." She was very discouraged but got her mojo back when she joined a family practice team in northern Labrador and was mentored by the six doctors of the team. "They taught me so much. Eventually, one said, "'I'm going on holidays . . .'"

"Don't tell me he asked you to cover for him!"

"An NP never covers for a doctor," Donna is quick to explain. "We don't replace physicians. We work together with them." But she emphasizes that an NP works differently than a doctor. "The way I practise is not about body parts, organ systems, or pathology. If a patient comes in with a headache, I do a complete exam. I talk to them about lifestyle, diet, exercise, stress. We have a *conversation*. No one gets past me without a conversation. At the end of the day, it's not rocket science to diagnose an ear infection, to treat someone's blood pressure, or to help them manage their medications. What people need most is to have a place to go, someone who will listen and care and will help them find what they need. NPs give people the primary health care they need and it reduces wait times. It's crazy, patients in the ER getting their ears syringed, blood pressure meds renewed, or foot care!"

Donna loves this population. "These are complex individuals, each desperately needing a holistic approach. You have to look at the whole picture. You can prescribe meds, but what if they can't afford them? You can order tests, but what if they can't get back for the results? It's about listening, observing, watching. Ninety per cent of your diagnosis comes from your assessment and asking questions – only 10 per cent from tests. I have to tease out the mental illness versus the behaviour, identify the main issues and what needs to be addressed first, and assess the level of the client's participation in their care.

"We treat a lot of at-risk youth. They're mad at the world. Behavioural issues. Substance abuse. Run-ins with police. Getting into trouble. Dropping out of school. Establishing trust is the most important thing."

"How do you do that?"

"By sitting, and asking questions, and then listening. You ask a question like, 'How was your childhood?' and magically, a door is opened. If they are using I say, 'You use for a reason. Perhaps it's to avoid the pain of something else in your life? We need to help you wean off the substance you're hooked on and start building a repertoire of other strategies.'" Donna leans in closer, with a secret to reveal. "Here's my belief. If there's a person in front of me struggling emotionally or psychologically, I'll say, 'When we don't get what we need at an early age, or we've been exposed to trauma like sexual abuse, abandonment, poverty, or violence, we grow up but our emotional self doesn't grow in sync. We stay stuck back there and there's catch-up to do.' It starts with forgiving themselves."

"Not the parent or the person who did them wrong?"

"Children always feel they are to blame. I tell them their parents could only do what they knew. They did the best they could. 'You will have to take over from here.' We try to help them get to the point where they can say, 'This happened, but now I can make different choices.'" She smiles at how much she loves her work. She's still smiling even when we compare salaries and discover she makes only slightly more than a full-time hospital RN in Toronto. "None of us went into this for the money," she says. "We'd be fools if we did."

Donna likes to solve puzzles. She tells me about a patient who came in with a shoulder injury – a dislocation. She ordered an orthopedic consult, but in the meanwhile, the patient also had pain from the elbow down. "I wondered if it was nerve pain from an impingement, so I imaged the elbow to check for an evulsion fracture – didn't want to miss that. 'Why did you x-ray the elbow?' the orthopedic doctor demanded. I never mind if my work is questioned. I like putting together the whole picture, coordinating the team and making sure everyone knows what is happening with the patient. I like preventing people from falling through the cracks. That is so satisfying." She sits back contentedly. "Yes, I do love this population," she repeats. "But, I have to admit, I love my patients wherever I am. I like to get to know people, not just fix their problems."

24

SOCKS AND CONDOMS

NURSE PRACTITIONER KATHY HARDILL takes a handful of condoms out of her backpack and approaches a young woman in thigh-high black boots standing on the street corner in front of a grocery store. She's teetering on high heels, wearing a black camisole, a lightweight windbreaker over her shoulders, and purple tights. It's twelve o'clock in the afternoon, but she's already hard at work. As Kathy told me at the start of our walk through the streets, parks, and back alleys of this town, "Sex work takes place around the clock, not just at nighttime."

"Do you need any condoms?" Kathy asks in a friendly, respectful way.

"No, I'm good. But thanks." She returns to scanning drivers. She's desperate to land an afternoon job, likely to buy a drug fix; as Kathy also explained, in this town, most of these women are selling their bodies for drugs. Kathy stands with her while she scans the oncoming traffic, chatting for a few minutes. She hands her a card for the 360 Clinic. "Come see us whenever you like."

"Whenever I think a woman is working, I ask her if she needs condoms," Kathy says as we carry on with our walk.

"It's a great icebreaker," I say as a joke, but I guess there's some truth to that. "How do you identify a woman who is working the street?"

"Many I have gotten to know individually, but they all work like her, walking slowly, scanning cars, searching for a man and trying to make eye contact."

Kathy Hardill is one of Canada's first "street nurses." She's an NP, teacher, researcher, scholar, and gonzo political advocate on behalf of the poor, homeless, and mentally ill.

"I'm taking you out on the street with me," she said, moments after we'd first met. We put on our boots and coats and headed outside.

"Are we driving?" I asked, turning toward the parking lot.

"No, we'll be taking bus number eleven." She made her two index fingers into ones, and motioned walking.

Now, as we walk along the sidewalk, heading for the centre of town, Kathy explains how she works. "I move around, learn the community, hang out with the people, get to know them. I make myself available, show them I'm approachable. I'll see them where they are, take care of them wherever they want me to – a crack house, a back alley, a parking lot, on a park bench. I go where the person is, rather than make them come to us. Clinics and appointments don't always work for them."

We trudge on through the snow, slushy in patches where the sun's rays fall. It has warmed up a bit today. Kathy notes that this increase in temperature – perhaps a harbinger of spring? – will make one less hardship for the homeless to endure.

Today Kathy is on the lookout for two individuals she's worried about. She'd like to offer one of them an intramuscular injection of penicillin to treat his STD.

"I try to make a plan with the person. I always say, 'If I take a test and the results are wacky and you need treatment, how am I going to track you down? Is there somewhere you go every day?' I won't take blood work or do any tests unless I believe the client will act upon the results." She checks a parking lot tucked behind a bank and a pet food store. "I'm sure I'll find him. If not today, then tomorrow."

The other person Kathy is looking for was cold and sockless last time she saw him. She wants to give him a pair of gloves and some warm wool socks.

"So many of the problems that homeless people have with their feet — like infections, blisters, frostbite — could be prevented by wearing dry, warm socks."

(I must bring this matter to the attention of my sock-knitting colleagues at the next meeting of the Bagel Club. Oh, how the yarn will flow and the knitting needles fly!)

"I always have socks to give out. Like the condoms, they're a way to help me engage with them. Socks and condoms also send the message that I'm all about keeping them warm and safe."

Every nurse has at least one patient — some have many — they carry around with them for the rest of their lives. I have mine. For Kathy Hardill, it was an art professor who lived in a shack with holes in the roof. Whenever it rained, the shack would flood with filthy water, complete with floating raccoon corpses. Once, the professor had to wade through the water to get to his precious paintings, which he tried to save as he moved from place to place. Eventually, he lost them all. Kathy's first nursing intervention was to get him a pair of boots. When she saw that he was limping and had a sore foot, she wanted to offer treatment, but he didn't care about his feet. "They're the least of my problems," he told her.

In addition to socks and condoms, Kathy hopes to soon hand out the new harm reduction kits that are currently in preparation. Before we left her office, Kathy had shown me a sample. It contained a set of multicoloured cookers, so each person can identify their own, filters, a tourniquet, needles, and little vials of sterile water for injection.

"You mean someone might shoot up with unsterile water, straight from the tap?"

"Or spit. Or puddle scum. Pickle juice. Toilet water. Whatever they can find. Thus the abscesses you've seen on people's arms," she says grimly.

I walk along beside Kathy, taking this in. We stop to enter a public toilet, both women's and men's; we check under a train trestle, looking for homeless people or working women. All the while, she's still searching for two people, scanning the streets and checking laneways and also telling me more about the risky business of sex work.

"It's indoors or outdoors, in all types of weather. It's men with mini-vans that have a baby seat in the back. It's guys from all walks of life." Kathy stops to check under the awning of a closed-up canteen used only in the summer. "It's dangerous work. There's even a 'bad date list.'" It's a confidential website where women can post licence plates, emails, telephone numbers, or anything that identifies bad johns.

Before we press on, Kathy opens her knapsack to show me what she carries: bus tokens, a few pairs of wool socks and gloves, vitamins, alcohol swabs, sterile syringes, lubricant, and condoms, including some flavoured ones, for oral sex. Condoms have huge currency on the street. The pimps control the number of condoms they give out and count them carefully so they know how many "jobs" each woman has done. Some girls are tempted to re-use them to keep some cash back for themselves and not have to hand over everything to their pimps.

With her kind, honest, concerned face, in jeans and a plain sweat-shirt, and her beat-up purple knapsack patched together by duct tape and hanging from her shoulder, Kathy is easy to trust, easy to like, easy to learn from, and I find myself doing all of these things every step of this walk. I marvel at the respect she conveys to a panhandler we encounter. She's a dishevelled woman with blackened teeth who comes up to us with grimy outstretched hands. Kathy digs into her pocket and hands her a loonie. She introduces herself and asks, "What's your name?"

"Sam. Got anymore? Got a toonie?" Sam gives forth a loud, wet, hacking cough.

Kathy has another loonie and hands it to Sam. "Here you go."

Sam gives them back. "D'ya have a toonie instead? I like them better than loonies."

"That's all I have for you today," Kathy says cheerfully.

I try to help. "Two loonies or one toonie – they both equal two dol-lars," I tell Sam. She doesn't think much of my arithmetic, but I try again. "They have the same value."

"Not to me," Sam says as she ambles off, coughing and spluttering as she goes.

We go where they are.

Just then, we're stopped by two high-school girly-girls in matching berets, candy-coloured gloves, and scarves. With their rosy cheeks, huge, pink, breathless smiles, and springy ringlets, they look like they're from another era. (Who wears ringlets, anymore?) Melissa and Jenny, it says on their "Jesus Christ of Latter-day Saints" name tags.

"Does faith play a role in your life?" Melissa and Jenny ask in unison, eager to save our souls.

I look up from my notes. "I'll let you field that one, Kathy."

Kathy is nicer than me. "Faith is definitely a part of my life, but I'm sorry, we don't have time to stop and talk with you now." Her rebuff is gentle but firm, in keeping with the peaceable way Kathy lives. She is in touch with nature, respectful of the wild. She and her husband kill the meat they eat so they know it's fresh, with no additives, hormones, or antibiotics and, most importantly, that it's been treated and killed ethically. "I want to know that it lived wild and free. I am going to honour it by having a say in how it's killed."

We walk on, stopping now and then to chat with various people who live on these streets, some Kathy knows and others she wants to get to know.

"What's a typical day like for you?" I ask.

"First, knowing there's no typical day. How can I itemize what I do? I'm investing in relationships that I don't know if I'll have or not. Sometimes you think you're doing one thing and it turns out you're doing another."

"I can feel how much you love your work."

"I like homeless people and people dealing with mental illness or substance abuse."

"Why?"

"Because no one else does. They're hungry, broke, confused, scared. Who would live this way if they had a choice? Who would be a drug addict if they had an alternative? That's why we start with, 'Okay, so you're a user. Let's start there. Are you using safely? Do you have clean needles? Are you rotating your veins? Are you injecting with the bevel of the needle facing up to preserve your veins? Are you heating the heroin adequately to dissolve the particulate matter, which can damage your veins? Are you doing what you can to avoid abscesses? Our clinic is your oasis of safety. We are your allies.'

"I meet people where they're at. If I hand you a clean needle, I'm telling you, 'You're important. I care about your health. If you don't care about your health, I will care about you until you are ready to care for yourself. When you want help, come and talk to me. I'll be there. Even if you're not ready to stop using there are other ways to treat your anxiety.' I'll do whatever it takes to start building a relationship. I want to convey the message that you're not a piece of shit. One guy told me, 'I'm a waste of skin.' 'Yes, you have problems,' I said, 'but you're worth investing in.' I told him he is like a one-hundred-dollar bill, torn and soiled, crumpled and tattered, but a hundred-dollar bill still has intrinsic value. 'That's you.'"

I can't imagine trying to get off a physiologically addictive substance like alcohol, cocaine, heroin, or cigarettes. I'm dealing with my own addictions — coffee, chocolate cake, for example. "Is meth a problem in this town?" I ask Kathy. (Clearly, I've been watching too much *Breaking Bad*, another of my addictions.)

"Not here. It's too expensive a drug for this population."

We arrive at a church drop-in centre and just before we go in, Kathy points out something across the street. There's a park with a gently sloping toboggan hill. At the bottom of the dip, at the base of each tree is a bale of hay, tied with a rope. "Put there to protect the kids, lessen the impact," Kathy notes dryly. "When I was a kid we learned to roll off in time."

The current trend of hovering parents and overprotected kids seems especially misplaced; I'm now meeting a lot of people who need more protection than our privileged children. I guess the bales of hay are a form of harm reduction, too.

As we enter the drop-in centre, we're hit with the smell of mashed potatoes and gravy. It would be a pleasant aroma if it were a homemade Thanksgiving dinner enjoyed with one's loving family around the dining room table; however, in this context, the smell is revolting. It doesn't help that it's mixed with the smell of cigarette smoke, body odour, and resignation.

The meal is being served in a crowded basement room, noisy with chatter, expletives, hoots of laughter, and the occasional loud exchange of harsh words. Hungry, dirty people sit at long metal tables, hunched over plates of food. We've just arrived and already I feel closed in. I'm sweating. Looking around the room, I see one exit. If I need it, I'll have to plow through this group of rowdy, sullen, or dejected-looking individuals to escape. They wear tattered or ill-fitting clothes and many have painful-looking piercings and scary tattoos like snakes or guns or barbed wire. Others just look down and out, angry or depressed. I swallow down my fear and copy Kathy's confident stride. Following after her, I enter the room boldly. In fact, I move past her, right into the midst of the people at the tables and those milling around the perimeter. I find a chair in the corner of the room and take out my notebook and pen; it's my standard retreat when I need to think, when I'm wondering about something and trying to understand it. In seconds, a man with spiders tattooed all over his face, a nose ring, and a black baseball cap clamped to his head comes over and leers at me.

"What are you doing? Are you writing something about me?"

I hadn't even considered how my usual activity might seem unusual in these circumstances.

"Why're you here?" he sneers. "Only retards come here." He moves in to look down at my notebook. There's no time to call out to Kathy for help. I tell myself to stay calm – or at least act that way. I look him in the eye, trying to think how I might connect with him, disarm him, bring down the tension.

"Why are you looking at me like that?" he shouts. He comes at me in a fury, his fists clenched. A friend of his jumps up and grabs his arm, saving me in time.

"Don't pay any attention to Kyle," the friend says, pulling Kyle away. "He's just pranking you. It's just that he's gone off his meds and is a little antsy."

I go over to Kathy, keeping my head up, though feeling I've failed a test. How could I ever win their trust if I were their nurse? I look too rich, too well fed. I wonder if she saw what happened.

She did. "You could waltz in here with a fur coat and diamond tiara. They wouldn't care."

The image of myself making an entrance in that attire makes me burst into laughter, releasing tension I'm still feeling from that close encounter with danger. Kathy continues, dead serious. "All they want is to be seen, to be acknowledged. They don't want you to pretend to know what their lives are like; they only want to know that you are willing to listen. Yes, they're watching you, checking you out, but it's not about what you're wearing or what you look like or what you have. They might tell you to fuck off, but if you stay, they know they can trust you. They want to know you're not judging them. It was good you made yourself at home and sat down." She looks at me approvingly. I feel better. Maybe I passed the test, after all.

"Were you frightened when that man lunged at you?"

"Yes, I was. A bit."

"I'd think you were disingenuous if you said you weren't."

We stand off to the side of the room. The way they are huddled together, squished on the benches, gulping down the soft, simple food makes me sadder than I've ever felt in the ICU. At least there, patients are being cared for. They have a roof over their heads and are hopefully getting some loving kindness from those of us caring for them. Out here, these people are all on their own.

"Every single person in this room has been hurt, abandoned, abused," Kathy says. "If you were to hear their stories you would not be able to fathom how they're still standing. When you see their suffering, and not just their bad behaviour, you feel enormous compassion."

Kathy points out one young woman who she says is a sex worker who uses crack cocaine. One day she told Kathy that her earliest memory is of her mother hitting her on the head with the stiletto heel of her shoe. She was prostituted by her pimp father, bounced from foster home to foster home, abused by —

"Okay, okay, I get it." I hold up my hands, cover my ears. I can't bear to hear anymore. I've reached my limit. "But what can you actually offer them?"

"We always want to see the results of our actions, but as a street nurse, you have to see the long-term benefits. You've got to be in it for the long haul — and I am."

As we leave the drop-in centre, she's pleased to find one of the clients she's been looking for, sitting outside on the stoop. "Hey, Brent, here you are," she says to an elderly man with a long white beard, wearing a Vancouver Olympics red-and-white toque. He's dangling his legs and we see there are no socks on his feet. Kathy hands him a pair of socks and a pair of gloves. "I'm glad I found you."

We walk on down to the river, where Kathy wants to check places where she thinks there might be more people, especially the other person she's scouting for. At the shore of the Ottonabee River, there's an inscription on a plaque that she stops to read: "I love history." In fact, she's quite a history buff. She's written an article about the history of street nursing in Canada, in which VON plays a big part. In addition to numerous "letters to the editor" and scholarly articles, she's written a report called *Under the Radar*, which examines the alarming incidence of substance abuse in rural areas and how it's often invisible and hidden. She tells me about a study that asked 454 homeless adults, "What is the hardest part about staying healthy when you are homeless?" She and her co-investigator hypothesized it would be "staying warm" or "finding food." They were shocked to discover the number-one response was "maintaining self-esteem" — expressed by one subject as "trying to feel good about myself when I get up in the morning."

"Powerful stuff, isn't it?" she asks.

We are walking back to the 360 Clinic now, but Kathy still hasn't found the person who needs an antibiotic injection; she plans to go out to look for him again later.

"And the woman you gave the loonies to is gone from her post, I see."

"Yes, Sam. She had a bad cough. I'll find her tomorrow. I want to listen to her lungs. Maybe I can coax her into the clinic for a checkup. I'll try to tempt her with a bowl of soup, a warm jacket, and a shower."

"A toonie might do the trick," I say. "Sam," I echo. I'd completely forgotten her name. Earlier, she was just another anonymous, beseeching face. Now I'm wondering where she is too. Does she have pneumonia, as Kathy suspects, and will she get treatment?

Back at the clinic, we sit in the office for a few more minutes to talk, drink coffee. I'm still trying to process all that I've seen today. "It's shocking how even the most terrible suffering can remain hidden," I say. "Most people can't even imagine there are people nearby living this way. I certainly didn't. It's unspeakably sad."

"And such unnecessary suffering. It doesn't have to be this way," Kathy says. She tells me that on any given night in Toronto alone there are at least five thousand homeless people, including the "hidden homeless," who are roving around, "couch surfing" from place to place each night. "It's a disgrace that we do not have a national strategy for poverty and housing." Shelters are only a temporary solution, she says. For her, the shelters with women and their children are the saddest because they perpetuate this legacy of suffering. Kathy compares homelessness to natural disasters like earthquakes and hurricanes, but homelessness is a serious human rights violation. "To have a home is a basic human right, along with health care, of course. That's why I couldn't do work downstream if I didn't work upstream, too."

"I've never really understood those terms."

"*Downstream* is service, *upstream* is advocacy. Working upstream makes an impact on a greater number of people. It's fighting for systemic changes through writing letters, signing petitions, lobbying politicians, making phone calls, taking reporters behind the scenes, as I've done many times. But I couldn't do the advocacy work if I wasn't on the scene, doing actual hands-on nursing care in the field."

Here's Judith's third type of nurse. Nurse Activist, Activist Nurse — consummate nurse.

Kathy wants to tell me a parable, and it's nice to relax and listen to a good story.

"There's a nurse who's tired. She needs a vacation. She goes fishing, enters the river in her hip waders, casts her line. Suddenly, she hears someone calling for help. She sees them struggling. They're drowning! So she rushes over, grabs the person, picks him up, and helps him clear his lungs. A nurse is never off-duty, as you know. But then, she sees someone else in danger. Another person is drowning . . . and then another and another. People are falling into the water and they don't know how to swim. Then the nurse figures if she builds a bridge and teaches water safety, maybe there won't be so many drowning victims. Instead of mopping up messes, the nurse also works on fixing the underlying problems."

Upstream, downstream. Now I get it. This fishing story will stick.

"Academics love theories. Here's my nursing theory: You take what you see in your daily clinical practice and allow that to inform what you do on a policy level or in the political arena. You can't do one without the other. They can't be separated."

When Kathy was living in Toronto, Canada's richest city, she worked in a men's shelter. There was an outbreak of tuberculosis that resulted in the death of three men. "We know that a shelter, or any crowded living space, is a breeding ground for infection, but tuberculosis? In this day and age, how can this be happening? TB is so preventable and treatable. We rallied together and called a meeting with the chief coroner. We marshalled our arguments, called for an inquest, and came forward, RNs and NPs, to testify as expert witnesses. That's an example of how downstream work leads to upstream work. But you'd need to be actually doing the work to know this."

And even when the challenges are as big as these, and there are so many problems she can't fix, Kathy stays true to a nurse's "North Star."

"We can always bear witness. Bearing witness is an important part of my practice."

I nod. "That's one of the reasons I write," I say, coming to this realization as I say it.

"We have access to people's hidden stories," Kathy says. "It's one of the great joys and privileges of being a nurse – to walk with people on their journeys."

I ask her the questions Judith asked me: "Why don't more nurses speak out on these issues? Why aren't they more politically active?"

Her response is more charitable and diplomatic than mine was a few months ago, when I first met Judith and got annoyed by this perfectly legitimate question.

"Most workplaces don't support nurses' involvement. They discourage it. Many nurses feel it's irrelevant or beneath them to get involved in politics to bring about change. They don't feel empowered to make speeches, to be vocal to politicians, attend rallies. They've been told so many times that their voices don't matter that they've begun to believe it. When I meet nurses who are intimidated or not empowered, I tell them to get over it. You are needed. There is so much to be done."

25

WORKING LIKE A DOG

I'M JUST ABOUT TO GET ON MY WAY when Krista, 360's office manager, suggests that, before I leave, I should stop by the adult day program located in the mall. "But I've already seen a few ADPs," I say. *If you've seen one, you've seen 'em all, no?* "But they're expecting you," she says with a twinkle in her eye. "There's a special guest today."

That's how I get to meet Bryce Balson, a retired forester, and Cody, his constant companion and a professional therapy dog.

"We usually come on Fridays," Bryce says. "Today's Thursday but we came to meet you. Cody knew it wasn't his day to work here." We look down at Cody, whose expression seems to say, *Of course I knew.* Cody is an old dog with the face of a young bear cub, and Bryce has the face of a gentle papa bear, covered in a ginger and grey beard. Bryce is a hardy outdoorsman in a flannel plaid shirt, suspenders stretched over a big belly, and a black baseball cap decorated with pins and yellow ribbons, reminders of soldiers stationed far away from home. He gazes down at his brilliant dog, who's sitting at his feet. "Cody's a Nova Scotia Duck Toller," Bryce says. "My granddaughter found him on the Internet. 'Here's a dog for you, Grandpa,' she said. He was scruffy, skinny, and his coat was dirty and matted like a bird's nest.

He'd been running the roads. But there was something about him, even though he wasn't looking his best that day."

He's certainly looking his best now. His coat is glossy and smoothly brushed. His shining eyes are locked on Bryce, reading his body, figuring out what is expected of him and then ready to spring into action. This dog has a strong work ethic.

"First thing, I had to make sure he was safe around children, so I asked a family with little kids if we could test him out. 'You can tell me to hit the road, if you want to,' I told them, but the closer the kids got, the more Cody wagged his tail. They pulled his ears and stuck their fingers up his bum, and he didn't flinch. Afterwards, he jumped into my truck right away. I chose him and he chose me."

"Do you think Cody knows he has a job to do?" I have the strongest sensation that he does and, as improbable as it sounds, that he's following our conversation.

"Seems to. When I took out his brush in the morning, he knew we were going to work."

If a dog can smile, Cody is smiling.

"He's pretty pleased with himself because we got past the 'no pets' sign today at the entrance to the mall. Once, we got stopped by the security guy. When I explained that Cody is a working dog, he seemed suspicious, but let us through. Another day, we got here early and Cody and I were walking around. This mall cop came to the VON office to complain. 'Why is that dog in the mall? Dogs aren't allowed.' I explained he's a therapy dog."

Just then, Buzz and Lorne, two participants in the day program, come over to meet me. Buzz, who's bald and looks exactly like Mr. Magoo, asks, "Didn't you play the trumpet with us in the Big Band?" I shake my head, no, as his buddy Lorne takes my hands and twirls me around. We do-si-do for a few steps, then he dips me down, ballroom style.

"Did Cody have to have any special training?" I ask, returning to them.

"The testing was *in-ten-sive*. They let him loose in a room with ten people walking, some with walkers or canes, each person making sudden noises. Cody didn't startle. Then they brought in a wheelchair – didn't fizz him in the least. Took a metal garbage bag with empty cans, banged on it. Put treats out to test that he didn't jump up and grab them or take them with his teeth. They even brought in other dogs to test for aggression. They put him through the paces and he came through with flying colours. Cody needed no training. He's a natural.

"People think any dog can do this work, but if the dog is skittish, or growly, it won't work," Bryce continues. "They have to have the right temperament to help people. There are dogs that guide blind people, fetch for people in wheelchairs, and ones that can detect a seizure coming on. The owner has to be trained as well as the dog. It's not as simple as people think it is. And it's not so simple to get a helper dog. One lady called me up to say, 'I've caught multiple sclerosis, can I get a dog to help me?' Did she think these dogs are party favours?"

Cody whimpers a little, and Bryce reaches down to pat his head.

On their days off, Bryce and Cody keep busy. They go to Highway 401, the portion of it called the "Highway of Heroes," where fallen soldiers are brought home in a procession. "That's why I wear yellow ribbons on my cap." He takes it off to show me. "It means 'you are not forgotten.' Cody and I go for each soldier, to pay our respects. There's no traffic and it's a cavalcade with a police escort and they slow down at the overpass. We wave our flags. No one talks, some people break down in tears. Oh, here comes Sister Anna."

Bryce and Cody share a glance. "Don't worry, Cody," Bryce tells him. "I'll be good. I promise. No dirty jokes when Sister Anna is around."

"I love Cody," says Sister Anna, joining us at the table. "Co-dy, Co-dy," she chants.

"One lady was scared," Bryce continues. "Imagine that. It took three months, but she patted him. 'That wasn't too bad,' she said. Soon she was patting him and calling him over.

"When people see Cody, it brings them out of their shell and they tell stories of their own pets. I can't tell you how many Spots, Rovers, and Fidos that Cody has reminded people of." Bryce gets up to bring us both a cup of freshly brewed coffee. I call Cody over to me, but he trots after Bryce into the kitchen and I follow them.

"You two are tied at the hip."

"Cody and I had never been separated, until last year when I had to go in for a five-artery bypass. It's a scary place, the hospital."

"Tell me about it," I groan. "I love it as a nurse, but as a patient? Not so much."

"So, one day last year my chest was paining me. The wife drove me into town and the doctor told me I needed an operation. Just before I went under, he asked me, 'Sir, do you have any concerns?' 'Yeah,' I said. 'Are you old enough to do surgery?' He looked like my teenage grandson. My little granddaughter said, 'You're sick, aren't you, Grandpa?' 'Grandpa's gonna come right,' I told her. 'You can't get married before you're twenty because I have to learn to dance first.' The first thing the doctor said when I woke up after surgery was, 'You'd better sign up for those dancing lessons, Mr. Balson.' I was still in the hospital and I had to see Cody, so they managed to wrangle an okay from the doctor to have him brought in. Did me a world of good. And didn't he go to work when he got there? We went room to room visiting patients, making them feel better. Cody is practically a nurse himself.

"One girl we visited was having a bad day. She was down in the dumps. Cody went to her. Seemed to understand she needed cheering up. He nudged her hand to get her attention. He doesn't usually lick people, but that day, he licked her hand. What a smile on her face. Cody reads people, he knows how they're doing.

"Cody's specialty is therapy, but I have read about a beagle named Cliff from Holland who sniffs human feces samples and can detect C. difficile bacteria with 99.8 per cent accuracy. He gets to sniff stool all day – what a sweet gig for a dog. I have a friend whose cat lets her know when her diabetic daughter's blood sugar is too low. In the dog park I met two dogs who work downtown detecting the presence of bed bugs."

Bryce knows of dogs who serve in the military, helping soldiers who come home from service with PTSD. "I know one bitch, if you'll excuse the term, who's high-strung, but when she's on duty, caring for a traumatized soldier, she dials it back and calms the guy down."

There is no doubt in my mind that Cody is listening to our conversation. He puts his head down on his front paws and heaves a contented sigh.

"Yup, Cody works hard. He also makes his rounds at the local retirement home. At first, it was like trying to herd cats. People were all over the place, wandering off in different directions. Cody comes from a long line of herders, but he soon realized he wasn't supposed to round up this crowd, nor bark or nip at their heels to bring them in line. At home he's frisky, but here, he's super-careful not to brush against anyone or get in anyone's way. Once, someone fell, and Cody went over to touch them on the nose to let them know someone was coming to help.

"He greets each person as they arrive, and if someone's sad or upset, or just having a bad day, Cody senses it. He goes over to lean into them and send them good vibes. He nuzzles them and stays close. He has his favourites, though, but he tries not to show it."

"What else does Cody like to do when he's not working?"

"Ordinary dog things – chase squirrels. Spooked a chipmunk the other day. It was chittering at him, right in front of him. Cody faked a lunge, deked him, and let out a bark. It worked. That chipmunk doesn't mess with Cody no more. You can learn a lot from a dog. Cody's an old dog, but he's still learning new tricks."

Bryce looks at Cody with love and Cody returns it.

26

FRIENDS WITH BOUNDARIES

"IF HE FINDS ME," she drops her voice and looks around furtively, "he'll kill me. Please don't use my real name."

Of course not, I assure her.

She takes a deep breath, looks me in the eye, and is ready to speak.

"More than one time, I have experienced the last few moments before death."

Even in her distress, Shahida remains articulate and beautiful, with dark, sad eyes and a smooth, perfect complexion. She sits in a booth at a suburban Tim Hortons, Nurse Allie Clinton at her side. She's frightened, cowed, but clearly wants to talk to me, to tell me what happened. The clothes she wears are in a style that's foreign to her. The blue jeans, high-necked sweater, oversized plaid shirt are uncomfortable; she's used to wearing a *hijab* to cover her head and neck, and a long dress with sleeves called an *abaya*, but her usual attire would make it easier to be recognized by someone from her Muslim community. Shahida needs to be unnoticed – ideally invisible – because she has gone into hiding. "That's why I'm wearing these Canadian clothes they gave me at the shelter." That's where she's staying after fleeing her husband, who tried to choke her. It wasn't the first time he'd attacked her, or the first time she'd tried to escape. But this time was different; she finally got away.

Shahida is a young mother of two from Pakistan who has lived in Canada for the past five years. "Shahida's home is not safe," Allie had explained tersely on the phone. "We can't meet there." She was careful not to say more, leaving it to Shahida to decide how much to disclose. But Shahida wants to talk. Before she begins, she warns me that what she is about to tell is "maybe 1 per cent of the story."

"My husband is a lawyer and he got a doctor friend of his to diagnose me with bipolar disorder." She pulls open a side pocket of the knapsack beside her to show me a plain, plastic red ring. "This key chain. It was the first thing. It was blue. He changed the colour to make me think I was losing my mind." Shahida wills tears not to fall from her eyes. "He told me I was crazy, unstable. '*Mental*,' he kept saying, and he'd slap the side of my head." Shahida smacks the side of her head to show me how he did it.

"When I met Nurse Allie at the shelter, I told her, 'I have bipolar, you know.'" She looks to Allie to tell her part of the story.

"When Shahida said that, something clicked in me," Allie recalls. "'Do *you* think you are bipolar?' I asked her."

"The way she asked my opinion validated what I believed deep down. That I wasn't crazy. He had me put on Valium, lithium, and other meds. I developed tremors and insomnia. I slept on the box spring; he slept on the bed. 'You're mental, mental, mental,' he kept saying. He told the kids, 'Your mother is mental.' I began to doubt myself. One day I asked him, 'Why do you call me mental?' 'Because you are crazy. I have no need for you, except for sex.'" She takes a deep breath and closes her eyes to calm herself before going on. "The credit card. That was the next thing. He left it on the kitchen counter. My son splashed water on it and bent it. That night I told him I needed a new one." She pulls the waterlogged credit card from her knapsack. "Here, I keep it to always remind me. He said, 'Imran didn't do this. You ruined it, so I'd have to get you a new one.' I was living with a man who didn't treat me like a human being. I sat like a statue for hours. Then, I went into the mosque and prayed for hours. The next day I went back and hid there, but he came and found me, and dragged me home. 'I want to go back to *my* home, to my parents,' I told him. 'You take the kids and I'll go.' But he'd hidden my passport. He told the judge I wasn't capable of being their mother, that I was unstable, had attempted suicide. I am crying now for the kids, but otherwise I am normal."

Her husband kept Shahida locked up at home, told the children's teachers that their mother was in a psychiatric facility. He hired two nannies to take care of the house and children.

"'Your words are killing me,' I told him. 'Your mother is crazy,' he told the kids. He hit me. Many times, he covered my mouth and nose, pushed me against the wall. That's why I always wear a turtleneck." She pulls it down to show me purplish-red streaks. "He made me keep my neck covered. A week ago he grabbed me by the throat. I tried to scream, but I couldn't. I pushed him back and ran to the bathroom and locked the door. *This is it. This is the time I will die.* I remember thinking that. Then I collapsed and blacked out for I don't know how long. When I woke up, I was still lying on the bathroom floor. He had gone to work and taken the kids to school. I took a cab to the shelter where I'm staying now. A friend told me about it. I had no money for a taxi and no idea where I was going. I'd only been out of the house a few times, just to go to the shopping mall. That's all he'd ever allow me."

Allie gives her money for lunch and while Shahida goes to the counter, Allie explains the odds against a woman escaping domestic violence. "It takes, on average, thirty-four assaults before a woman finds the courage to get out. Most don't."

It takes twenty pounds of pressure to flip the tab on a can of soda, and only a few more to occlude the trachea. I remember Morag's research on strangulation.

Allie has been visiting Shahida in the shelter every day and will accompany her to a psychiatrist to assess competency, as well as to the custody court to bolster her courage and make sure her voice is heard.

Making sure her client gets heard is challenging because, as Allie muses, "I don't think I ever realized the extent to which the medical and legal systems can be influenced by culture, especially dominant patriarchal ones. Shahida and I will be navigating together through this frightening labyrinth. I want to make sure she is seen and her voice heard."

"Nurse Allie is my lifeline," Shahida explains, returning to sit with us, a sandwich in hand. "I couldn't go through this without her."

"You are social worker, lawyer, and therapist, too," I say to Allie, "as well as nurse."

"Nursing puts the pieces together. I want to bring everyone to the table and make sure Shahida has choices. I'm the constant, ensuring everyone knows the story and stays on track."

"Nurse Allie gave me hope," Shahida says. "She was the first one who saw me as possibly sane. What I've told you is just bits and pieces," she says, thanking me for the opportunity to share even that. "Maybe it will help some other woman to get out like I did."

Finally! Thanks to the sympathetic ear of my friend Annie's nurse manager, and her willingness to slice thorough the bureaucracy for me and expedite the process, I've been given permission to go on visits with four nurses who work for Toronto Public Health. That's how I got to meet Allie. I'll now spend an hour or two with Annie, and then accompany the other nurses tomorrow. These nurses all work with new mothers, and I'm here to watch Annie teach young women how to connect with their babies. "I wish I'd had someone like me when I had my babies," she says.

"I do, too," I agree.

Annie works with young mothers who are poor, new to the country, or struggling in some way. "If you're young and have a baby, I want to support you to be the best mom you can be," Annie says, her practical intelligence showing through her lighthearted tone.

We drive to a strip of row houses in downtown Toronto. Her first client of the day is a young mom named Rita, a tall, attractive nineteen-year-old with long dark hair, holding a squirming baby on her hip.

Today, Annie is here to talk with her about baby safety. She explains that the baby might go into unsafe places. "As his mother, you are there to protect your baby. You have to decide whether to keep your eye on him constantly or make sure your home is always safe and clean so you don't have to worry."

Rita thinks this over, putting visible effort into showing interest in what Annie is saying. "I still can't believe I'm even a mother," she says as she sets Darwin, her ten-month-old bright-eyed baby boy, down on the carpet in front of her. Annie gives her a toy to hand to Darwin, and, when cued, Rita does that. Annie helps Rita figure out which option she prefers, constant vigilance or baby-proofing. Together, they plan a strategy to make this small, stuffy studio apartment safe for Darwin on Rita's minimal budget.

"At six months, babies don't know the word 'no,'" Annie explains, "so you must keep the home safe." Rita does not look pleased with the work that baby-proofing entails. She sighs wearily.

Annie gets down on all fours and suggests that Rita do the same so that she can see Darwin's world as he sees it. "That's the best way you'll be able to tell what your baby can get into and what may not be safe for him."

"My son's baby-daddy left me during the pregnancy." Rita sits back up to explain her situation to me. "He doesn't give me money, never tells me if he's going to visit the baby. He left while I was giving birth, came back a few days later, then left again."

Annie fills in the rest. Rita had to be admitted to the hospital for psychiatric treatment for a few weeks. Her brother and sister took care of the baby during that time. We watch Rita play with her baby in the ways that Annie has taught her and has rehearsed many times.

I ask Rita about her family. "They try to be good to me, but I don't trust them. I prefer to stay away from them, indoors alone, by myself."

"You're not alone now. You have Darwin to look after," Annie reminds her.

Rita nods. "My family is very educated but they keep reminding me about my schizophrenia and nagging me to take my meds. Part of me doesn't believe I have this thing, but it's also a relief to think I have it and that it's not my fault that I have a thing that affects my judgement."

The baby's father's absence is the matter that seems to vex her much more. "He comes over but won't bring any diapers and won't look after the baby. Sometimes I feel scared when he's over. But I promised Annie I'd tell her if there's a problem. Annie has helped me a lot. She tells me what to expect, and how to play with Darwin, how to teach him. When I ask her questions, her answers are not just fluff, they're scientific. I couldn't manage without her."

"It's about *attachment*," Annie says. "It's the most important thing for mother and baby." Establishing daily routines, for example, fosters attachment. They give the baby a sense of security. Annie gets down on the floor with Rita and they play with Darwin. Annie coaches her, whispers cues, suggests gestures, words that seem to still feel deliberate and awkward to this young mother. She teaches Rita how to play Follow the Lead, a game in which the baby is in charge and the mother mimics whatever the baby does, talking to him all the time, but letting him have the feeling that he's in charge. "Be a mirror for your baby," Annie says.

Rita picks up Darwin with the attention you'd pay to a bag of groceries and takes him into the kitchen as if to unpack rather than feed him. Annie and I stay behind for a few minutes to allow her to get set up and so that we can talk.

"I never play with the baby myself. It's very important that a mother doesn't even once see him reacting more with me than her. She might lose her confidence. For some of the women I work with, you, the nurse, might be the first person who they can trust, possibly the only one."

Annie has come to realize that *trust* may have different meanings to different people. "I had a challenge caring for one mother. I felt she didn't trust me. 'Of course I trust you,' she said, 'I let you into my house, didn't I?' Her definition of trust was not the same as mine. She was from a totalitarian, war-torn country that had been invaded, where citizens had no rights and the police could enter at any time. Allowing a stranger into her house was, for her, the ultimate sign of trust."

As we wait for Rita, I look around the room. There is a plastic house, a wooden train, and a few stuffed animals. I remember the expensive baby paraphernalia I had, the mounds of shiny new gadgets and gizmos my friends and I bought for our babies — or was it for ourselves?

"This is good. Some mothers have *no* toys for their baby," Annie says. "Each home you go into is a different world. In one, there may be so much dirt and clutter you can't even see the floor, it's stuffy and hot, the baby is overdressed, finances are limited, but the mom is confidently breast-feeding. Another single mom — upscale neighbourhood, the mother is anxious, isolated, having postpartum depression. Baby is dressed nicely. He gives a little holler, she panics. Behind each door, you're swept into a different world. Some places there's so much stuff, you can't see the floor. It's so hot and close. Mom is clutching the baby, won't put him down. She's freaked out, anxious. The place smells musty and mouldy. It's not healthy, but you can only deal with one thing at a time."

Annie looks mildly discouraged about today's visit with Rita. Knowing Annie as I do, I'm sure she'd like to deal with a lot more than one thing, but she knows her top priority. "What I really need to do is instil in a mother a sense of the importance, the significance of this baby. A baby is a big deal! I'm not sure Rita sees it that way."

Annie is concerned about Rita and her baby, but recognizes the limitations of her role. "All we can really deal with is the here and now, the basics like play, bonding, feeding. My expertise is fostering the bond between them by helping her get into her baby's mind. It's a skill that can be learned and is the first building block for empathy. Empathy — even for one's own child — does not come naturally to everyone."

Rita brings her baby back in and sits with us. She's stiff and uncomfortable with him, holding him like he's an inanimate plastic doll. She seems bored or disinterested in playing any more with Darwin.

Back in Annie's car, I think of that image — it's the picture of *detachment.*

Annie and I talk about words.

"They are so important." Annie says. "There was one, a twenty-year-old Cambodian mother with a five-year-old son. He was completely dysmorphic, with no speech. I could see she had no idea how disabled her son was. 'He's lovely. You are doing a wonderful job,' I told her. Her entire body eased with relief. 'I thought his not speaking was my fault,' she said. That opened the door for us to talk about his special needs. I didn't use the word 'disabled.'"

"It must be tempting to bring them toys. Rita had so few. I had so many when my kids were little. Too many." I wonder if I could drop off those toys for Annie to give to Rita.

"Unfortunately, we can't. No, it harms the relationship if we move too far over into friend mode. I use my *self* in my practice. Sure, I'm warm, genuine, and caring, but there is a boundary that I never allow myself to cross. Sometimes they'll push a button or two of mine, but only I'm aware of it. I don't let on. We are friendly, but we have to be clear about boundaries."

Public Health Nurse Talia Singer also works for the City of Toronto. She's involved with a program for pregnant women living on the street, called HARP (Homeless At Risk Prenatal program). We're in the heart of downtown, walking to meet Kaitlin, a twenty-four-year-old cognitively impaired woman who gave birth to a baby girl two weeks ago. Talia is bringing a bag of groceries and toiletries to give to Kaitlin. "No one ever discharges a new mother from the hospital with maternity pads." It's one of Talia's pet peeves, so she always puts it on her shopping list for her clients, along with groceries, food vouchers, bus tickets, and phone cards, all subsidized monthly expenditures for the young, homeless mothers Talia sees. As for the cellphone, Talia explains: "They need them. They may be homeless, but at least they're connected. On average, I get over two hundred texts per month, per client. Sometimes they lose their phone or sell it for food or crack."

Talia's puffy winter jacket hides her compact figure and her curly chestnut hair is casually tousled. She is naturally pretty, but her good looks don't seem to matter to her in the least. She's been a nurse for twelve years, but is as fresh and enthusiastic as a new grad. As we tramp through the snow and city grime to get to a coffee shop, Talia explains that this baby Kaitlin recently gave birth to is her fourth, all with the same partner. Each time, the Children's Aid Society has intervened and taken the baby, because Kaitlin and her partner, who's currently out on parole on a charge of assault, have neither a home nor the skills to parent. "Kaitlin is upset because her doctor is pressuring her to get a tubal ligation to prevent further pregnancies."

I stop short. "That sounds like a good idea." I assume I'm stating the obvious, responding how anyone would after hearing even a snippet of that background, but Talia visibly bristles at my endorsement of the doctor's advice. "You don't agree?" I ask in disbelief.

"No, I don't. Enforced sterilization in this country is illegal and unethical. It's what oppressive regimes do, what the Nazis did to non-Aryans. It is used for ethnic cleansing."

"But Kaitlin is homeless, cognitively impaired. She doesn't have a stable partner."

"Perhaps with the proper supports in place, Kaitlin could be a good mother. That's what she wants. She wants to keep her baby."

"I want to win the lottery, but that's not going to happen."

"If you'd been there in the hospital the day Kaitlin gave birth, and saw how she looked at her baby with love, you might feel differently. If you heard her wails when her baby was taken away, you'd feel her desire to be a mother. Kaitlin barely speaks, but that day, she made her voice heard. Who are we to destroy her dreams?"

"We're supposed to nurse people's dreams, too?"

"We all have dreams. She has the same dreams as you and I do. My job is to be on her side. She has no one else." Talia is clear about her role, which still seems ambiguous to me.

"What if her wishes are unreasonable? Harmful? Irresponsible?"

"Obviously, I don't support those, but I will agree to help her make healthy choices. That can only happen if she trusts me. All of this is about building a relationship. In my role we look at strengths. Her partner, Slade, has not been violent to her, they are not hard-core drug users, they want to be good parents."

Talia is younger than me by at least twenty years but suddenly seems wiser and more mature. Why can't I be as accepting and open-minded as she is?

"You must think I'm not very compassionate," I say.

"No, I don't. You ask the same questions my husband asks, that everyone asks."

"Welcome to my office," Talia says. In this bustling Tim Hortons, taxi drivers, university students, biker boys, and skater dudes stand in line for coffee and doughnuts. The language of the customers in front of the counter and of the servers behind is a mix of Hindi, Farsi, Jamaican patois, and Korean. The place is packed. No smoking is allowed, but it's hazy inside and reeks of cigarettes and the city.

Soon Kaitlin and Slade arrive. They're angry – he more than she – that their visit with their baby was cancelled because the foster parent was unable to bring her. They dig into the egg salad sandwiches Talia had bought for them. They huddle together, close to the table, warming their fingers around the paper cups of the "double-double" coffees she knows they like. Kaitlin's running shoes are covered in snow and her once-white-now-grey thin ski jacket doesn't look very warm. Slade wears a soaking wet black jacket and sports an earring.

"I'll negotiate an extra visit with your baby for you." Talia makes a reminder to herself.

They cheer up at that, especially Slade. "We'll get her back one day," he assures Kaitlin, who's staring at the rack of doughnuts, seemingly transfixed.

I try to imagine these two as parents – I can't. I decide I'll just try to put all judgement aside so that I can be as open-minded and sympathetic as Talia is. I will do my best not to allow myself to think of this baby's likely bleak future growing up in foster care. I make myself stop wondering

how the couples I know who desperately want a baby but who struggle with infertility would feel about this. I push out of my mind the protest of taxpayers over assuming the cost for people who produce children they are unable to care for, not to mention the children themselves without a permanent home who might or might not become adopted. I force myself to stay in this moment and attempt to keep my heart as open as Talia's is; I'm going to do my best to see what she sees without evaluating it.

"Maybe we could get more visits," Kaitlin wonders. *Crullers, dutch-ies, old-fashioned, sour-cream glazed.* "The driver didn't show. We didn't get to see our baby." *Maple iced, jelly, chocolate dip.*

"Hey, can you please make Kaitlin wash down there. I keep telling her that if you don't clean it, it'll get infected."

"Do you have discharge, Kaitlin? Is there a smell?"

"It smells and it still hurts. You know, the place where I make pee-pee."

I wonder if she is referring to her vagina or her urethra and if she knows the difference.

Slade leans forward in earnest. "I don't want her to get an infection. Hey, did you tell Talia about your milk?" He grabs her breast and squeezes.

"All gone." She holds up her hands and giggles.

Slade updates Talia about his battle with law enforcement. "They want me to go to anger management. They say I can't control my temper. There was a knife assault, but they want me to plead guilty, but I'm not going to plead guilty for something I didn't do, even though it would only be thirty days."

"What'll you do if Slade goes to jail?" Talia asks Kaitlin. "Where can you go to get food?"

While Kaitlin thinks that over Slade tells us his pre-jail plan. "Before I go back in – if I have to – I want to buy her a big pillow, shaped like a heart. For Valentine's Day." He whispers this as an aside so Kaitlin won't hear. No worry about that, her attention is elsewhere.

Somehow, Talia gently manages to bring the conversation around to birth control.

"We still want a baby," Kaitlin reminds Talia, in case she forgot.

"Yes, but for now, you need to give your body a rest. How about an IUD? It won't protect you from STDs, but you two are in a solid relationship."

She giggles, then pretends to pout and points a finger at Slade. "Sometimes he cheats."

"No IUD," Slade says. "I won't have no plastic thing bouncing off my you-know-what."

"This takes effect immediately. You don't have to wait thirty days like with the pill."

"We never did wait no thirty days last time." He grins at Kaitlin.

"I will bring you one next time and show you how it works. You can decide together."

"My doctor wants me to get my tubes tied. I'm not going to do that." Kaitlin stamps her foot. The snow has melted and her soaking wet shoes make squishing sounds under the table.

Slade nods his head in agreement. "Nope. She's not going to do that."

"It's your decision. It's your body. Okay, so what are you two going to do today?"

"Get some groceries. We'll go to the food bank. Then get high." Slade sees something over at the counter that puts a scowl on his face. He nudges Kaitlin and points at two police officers standing in line for coffee, but she doesn't get his drift.

"At the food bank, you don't get to choose what you want," she complains.

"What do you feel when you see the cops, Slade?" I ask.

"I hate them. All's they want to do is make my life a living hell." He stands up abruptly, suddenly eager to split. "Well, I guess I inhaled that food," Slade says. "Let's go, Kaitlin." He tugs at her jacket sleeve to move her along but Talia has more to discuss with them.

"You know," she says. "When we're not meeting anymore, there will be no more food vouchers. How will you eat? You texted me that you're only eating macaroni. Why is that?"

Slade shrugs in answer, glancing again at the police officers, then at the door.

Kaitlin giggles. "I don't like the food bank. They just give you stuff. I don't want tuna."

"How are you managing with money?"

"We get $677 a month. After phone, food, and rent there's twenty bucks. That's for weed. I need that." Slade folds his arms across his chest. "I need my weed. It keeps me calm."

"Slade calm is a good thing." Talia chuckles and pats him on the shoulder.

"I need some weed, right now." He's restless, shifting around in his seat. "I'm pissed because my lawyer says I have to do thirty days, but no, I have enough stress with the kid taken away. We have an empty stroller, an empty crib. I can't do time now."

"I put lotion on the baby," Kaitlin pipes up. "I even got peed on."

"You're parents. You're going to get peed on, puked on."

"We know what to do," Slade says. "Feed her, change her."

Just give me the keys to the car, Mom. I know how to drive.

"But we can't play with her yet. She's too small for that," Kaitlin agrees.

"Yes, she's only three weeks old. You can't play with her but you can talk to her and smile at her." Talia checks her calendar. "Kaitlin, we have a month left together. What can I help you with?"

She squints back at the pastries in a way that makes me think she might need glasses. Slade shifts around in the chair, drums on the tabletop. "We need to move on. C'mon Kaitlin." He tugs at her sleeve again.

Talia asks Kaitlin directly. "What can I help you with?"

They both stare back at her.

"What do you need right now, Kaitlin?"

She licks her dry, inflamed upper lip. "Chapstick."

"Don't lick it." Slade slaps her hand playfully. She puts her fingers to her lips. "Stop picking at it." They stand up to leave. Kaitlin's coat flaps open to her still-swollen belly.

"When our visits end, I will give you names and numbers of people who can help you."

"Can I still text you?" Kaitlin asks.

"Of course." Talia is about to say goodbye, but Slade is not as anxious to rush back into the cold now that the police officers have left the coffee shop.

"You don't have to say goodbye, Talia. You'll be seeing us again. Maybe even nine months from now. We have a plan, right Kaitlin? Let's tell her."

Talia is bemused, interested to know what these two are planning. Me, too.

"We're gonna keep on having babies until they let us keep one." He grins at Kaitlin.

"It's a plan," she says, high-fiving him.

This plan drops on me like a bomb, exploding in my mind. *I've lost my sympathy; I have no more compassion.* I turn my back on them in my mind. *Lucky they didn't try to high-five me!*

It astounds me how casual and easy is the act that results in something as monumental and significant as a new human life. I realize that now in a way I never have before.

Talia is nonplussed. She reminds Kaitlin how difficult her last pregnancy was, especially when she went into labour. How she had to use her last taxi voucher to get to the hospital the night she had early contractions. At the hospital, they told her it was false labour and they sent her off by herself with no taxi, coat, or boots, at two o'clock in the morning. She had to walk home, nine months pregnant. Somehow she got back to the hospital the next day, and when she had the baby, they kept her for twenty-four hours, then sent her home. Nine stitches, no maternity pads, no food, no home to go to.

"I'm going to miss you two." Talia gets up to give them each a hug.

Talia looks at me. She senses I'm struggling to process all of this. "Maybe next time Kaitlin gets pregnant she'll remember our good interaction and seek out a public health nurse."

"Being pregnant garners them a lot of attention. Maybe they should get this kind of attention for not getting pregnant," I suggest, trying to come up with a *solution*. "Don't you worry that your supportive approach might be enabling their bad choices?"

"But the alternative – advice, judgement, scolding criticism, punishment – will only alienate them. Then we'll lose them altogether. They need love." Talia smiles contentedly, like the Buddha I'm beginning to think she actually is. "Slade has a nurturing side, doesn't he?"

"An angry side, too." I shudder to think how he'll deal with the terrible twos.

I'm trying to figure out if Talia is preternaturally wise and extraordinarily compassionate – even saintly – or if she is merely naïve and incurably optimistic?

"What will happen after you discharge her from your care?"

"I will try to connect Kaitlin to adult protection services and other community agencies that assist people with special needs. I hope she goes but she may not. She's rejected it before. There is a trustee in charge of her who gives her an allowance from her family."

"I have a feeling you're going to be worried about them."

"It's hard for her when Slade is incarcerated. He's good at finding food for them."

"What does he do to get food?"

"Who knows? They eat."

Talia sees my shock at the way she nurses this client.

"It must seem that what I do is mothering or being a girlfriend. I am her nurse and she's my client. The boundaries are definite and clear to me. And Kaitlin is an adult and is entitled to make her own decisions. I will never try to take that away from her."

Who am I to say they can't be suitable parents? Perhaps Talia is right. They could learn, couldn't they? Who are we to quash their dreams? It's not money, intelligence, or education that makes for a good parent, is it? No, but it takes more than love.

"Do you have certain goals with a client like Kaitlin?"

"My goal is to establish a good relationship with her."

"Okay, so let's say you have that good relationship, then what?"

"A safe delivery in a hospital, not on the street."

"Yes, but she can walk into any hospital and be assured of safe care."

"Yes, but she might choose not to go to a hospital and have her baby in some unsafe place. She's felt disrespected in hospitals. Homeless people dread the hospital. They feel hostility from the staff. They feel disrespected, put down."

This seems to be a common theme. We seem to have a bad rep.

"I know in the hospital you like things you can fix." I nod at that. "Out here, there is no fix, only the hope that maybe, just maybe, if I take care of the mother, she will be better able to take care of her baby." She knows I'm skeptical. "Look, I don't know if this approach is right or wrong, good or bad, helpful or not. It's just about taking an interest in them and their story."

But as nurses we want to be *useful, too.* We're practical people. We can't just sit here, we have to *do* something. But what Talia is saying — and showing — is the opposite: It's more like, don't just *do* something, *sit* there. But then I consider it from another angle. What if Talia weren't in their life? Kaitlin and Slade would have nobody, they'd be cut off from society altogether. I understand what Talia does, and appreciate its importance, when I think of its absence.

"Remember when you were first pregnant and so excited? Well, I'm the one being excited for her. When her baby was born, she looked at him with absolute love. She wants to be a good mother. She howled when they took her baby away. That sound will stay in my head. Forever."

"How do you cope emotionally with this job?"

"Nothing stops the images, the voices, but my life is happy. I have a wonderful family. I am studying to become an art therapist."

"Have you ever been in a situation where you felt threatened or unsafe?"

"The surroundings may be scary, but not the people."

"What about rats? Seen any?"

"Oh, lots of rats," Talia says with a laugh. "Bed bugs bother me more because you can carry them home. They take over your house, get into the walls. They bite, cause infections, and they are hard to get rid of."

"What's your measure of success?" There has to be quantifiable results or objective metrics. What about outcomes? You need these things, especially in these days of fiscal restraint and having to account for every expenditure, don't you? It's a stretch for me to abandon my thirty years of pragmatic, problem-solving hospital training.

Talia tells me about one evaluation method that involves examining client text messages. There is plenty of data. One month, Talia received 263 texts from one client alone – and she has twelve clients at any given time. They track the frequency and content of the texts to examine them for research purposes.

"What do they text you about?"

"Appointments, questions, chit-chat." She scrolls down to show me a sampling from one client.

"I felt it kick."

"I'm in pain."

"Funky smell from my vagina."

"Do you think they'll take this baby away, too?"

"Sometimes they text me to disclose something like 'I'm using.' Or 'I'm high.'"

"How do you respond to that?"

"Always the same thing. Thank you for telling me. I'm honoured by your trust."

She shows me a back-and-forth exchange with one client:

"No epidural ☺"

"It's a girl. Emily. Five pounds, two ounces."

"*Congratulations!*"

"My BP is high. 24 hours and they're kicking me out the door."

"Where are you going?"
"Back to shelter."
"How are you getting there?"
"Taxi."
"What about the car seat?"
"Yup. Put in taxi. ☺"

"It sounds like two besties," I say.

Talia clarifies the relationship. "We're professional friends. Friends with boundaries."

In this kind of nursing, the personal and the professional could become so intertwined and enmeshed, but Talia knows what she's doing; she is clear about her boundaries and what she offers and what she doesn't.

"Developing a relationship with the mother is the only thing I can do that will make a lasting, positive effect," she says serenely. "Here, our successes are different. They're difficult to measure or even describe."

From the outside, Humewood House looks like an old-fashioned English boarding school, but not the magical Hogwarts variety, more the grim, institutional type. The inside is warm and inviting, and the women at the reception desk are expecting us. This is a group home where pregnant teens receive prenatal care, have their babies, and stay for up to six months after they give birth.

Since graduating from nursing school five years ago, Nurse Debi Wade has worked in labour and delivery and in a neonatal ICU. Recently, she started working for Toronto Public Health. "I wanted to know how they are doing after the hospital. When the mother and baby go home," she explains.

"This teen shelter is nicer than most. One place downtown has picnic tables. It smells old and dirty and there are broken-down couches, women always slumped in them, sleeping it off."

Many of the girls in Humewood House are in high school. That's why it's so quiet, the director told us. Right now, some are studying for midterm exams. We wonder what is taking Debi's client, DeShae, such a long time to come down after we called up to let her know we're here. We wait in the communal living area where there is nice pseudo-antique furniture and upholstered, slightly frayed couches. After about ten minutes, she appears, looking drowsy and indifferent to our visit. She places a box of Ritz crackers she'd been carrying under her arm, along with a sketch drawing on a scrap of paper of little pink hearts surrounded by blue tear drops, onto the coffee table in front of us. She sits down on a faded, floral wing chair and stares blankly ahead.

"Looks like you just woke up," Debi says, standing up to greet her.

DeShae slips off her moccasins, folds her tall self into the chair, and tucks her bare feet under her. Snuggling in deeper, she yawns broadly. Her tiny belly bulges slightly under her midriff top. She's skinny and pretty, with even features, straightened hair with extensions falling to her shoulders in waves, and long, purple fingernails. I can imagine her getting dolled up for prom night, and how much she'd probably love to be doing just that. She pulls out her phone and holds it close, resting it on her tiny baby bump.

"So, did you, DeShae?"

"Did I what?"

"Just wake up?"

"I like to be called Victoria, I mean Chloe." She starts humming a song under her breath. I instantly recognize Rihanna's "Diamonds."

"So, how's it going here at Humewood House?" Debi asks.

Chloe echoes Debi's earlier comment: "This place is nice compared to others I've been in." She rests her face in her hand, picks up her phone, and wipes the screen with the back of her forearm. She looks at it — not to make a call, but to use the screen's reflection as a mirror so she can fix her eye makeup and pick sleep out of the corners of her eyes.

Debi gets to the point. "Do you have any questions about your pregnancy? Any questions about the baby? Let's see . . . you're at twenty-three weeks. How are you feeling?"

"Kinda good." Chloe repositions herself, rearranges the cushions behind her back.

"Do you have any discomforts?"

"Just pressure, pain."

"Where?" Debi asks and Chloe looks away. "In your lower back?"

"No, in my neck." She won't meet Debi's eyes.

"Is she stoned?" I mouth to Debi, who shakes her head, no. To me she looks and acts that way, but Debi had told me they are very strict about their no-drug policy here, and she hasn't heard any complaints about her so far. Debi goes through a list of symptoms like nausea, vomiting, headaches, leg pains . . . Chloe shakes her head no for each one.

"How did you get here to Humewood House? How did you hear about it?"

"A friend of mine told me. She got pregnant and stuff in middle school and came here."

"Where is your family? Why are you not at home?"

"I came from a group home. I was in foster care. I'm a good kid. I didn't get into trouble, but when I got pregnant I couldn't stay there no more. Anyway, Imma be eighteen soon and can't stay there no more." She runs down the rest of her bio like a practised drill. "Seventeen years old. Came to Canada at ten. Born in Haiti – but I tell people Barbados, where Rihanna is from." She continues. "Foster care since birth. Group home since the age of thirteen. Mother dead. Father in jail back in Haiti. Four brothers, three sisters, no contact with any of them."

"Do you have friends from the group home?" Debi asks gently.

"No. I mean they're nice girls and stuff, but I don't want to bug them with my problems. Besides, they're younger than me." She looks down at her belly with surprise. "She's moving."

"Do you like that?"

"It's annoying sometimes but at least I know she's not dead."

"It's a good sign," Debi says. "About two or three movements an hour."

Chloe looks at her belly like it belongs on someone else's body.

"If it's not moving you should tell someone."

"Why?" She stares off into space. "She's still moving . . . stopped now."

Debi takes a different tack. "So, you know it's a girl?"

Chloe stares off into space. She looks bored. "It's moving . . ." She looks excited. She looks dismayed. "Stopped now."

"Are you comfortable staying here? Do you like it?"

"At my group home they don't lock everything up like they do here. The rules here are too strict."

"Yes, you do have to follow them if you want to stay."

Chloe is quiet.

"Do you want to stay?" After a long silence, Debi asks again, "Are you planning on staying here?"

"I'll try my best. They won't let me back in the group home cuz I'm pregnant. Here, at least, you get an allowance and there are one-, two-, three-, or four-dollar chores. I only want the four-dollar ones. Why should I work for less than that? But those ones get snapped up fast."

Every few minutes her mood shifts, from disinterest to defiance, from anticipation to disenchantment, from excitement to apathy; a tiny peak of interest, then it drops off.

She pokes her belly. "Best part about being here? I have my own room. I'm doing grade nine math, grade ten English. I had some rough patches at school cuz I didn't always have a bus ticket to get there. My older sister beat me up and stuff, so I had to go into foster care, but I ran away. I rode back and forth on the subway, but then it closes at two in the morning. One night they called the police."

"How old were you?" I ask.

"Fourteen. Foster family was okay and stuff. Better than at my mom's."

"What about the baby's father?"

"He wanted me to get an abortion. So I went to a clinic. Even signed the papers, but something told me to wait. I changed my mind. It's against my religion. 'You don't know what you're getting into,' he said.

'The baby will cry. You won't be able to finish school.' He already has a kid, with another girl." She looks at us like she knows what we must be thinking.

"We didn't use a condom because I thought he was the one. I wanted him to be my baby's daddy and more. I was hoping it wasn't just a booty call with him, it was a real relationship. I thought he'd be my hubby, not just my baby's daddy."

"Does he know you have decided to have this baby?"

"Yes, and he promised he'd be there for me. He said, 'If you get pregnant, I'll support you,' but now he says 'sorry' and disappeared. We argued too much. He didn't want to spend New Year's with me. He spent it with her. Now I want him out of the picture." She wipes away a tear. "We haven't spoken for a long time. Maybe three days."

"Does he know you're here?"

"Don't know. I texted his mother. She said she'd be here for me, but she's never even come to one doctor's appointment. She has a car, so there's no excuse. I thought I had a good relationship with her. I never disrespected her. She's wish-wash."

"So when you go to your appointments, does someone go with you?"

"No, I go alone. I definitely learned my lesson. I won't get into this situation again."

"How do you feel about going through this pregnancy?"

"Bad. I wanted a boy. It's a girl. She hasn't anything good to face. I have to have this baby. I don't have a choice."

"Sometimes, a mother decides to give her baby up for adoption."

"That's crossed my mind, but I don't think I could handle it." A tear drops down onto her lap. "I can't imagine giving away a baby that I carried inside me."

"We can talk more about this," Debi says. "Chloe, do you feel depressed?"

"I never thought this is how my life would turn out. I didn't think I'd get pregnant. I had five months of unprotected sex and didn't get pregnant." She sniffles and looks down, not at her belly, but the floor.

"How do you see your future? Do you plan to finish high school? If you do, it's very possible for you to meet that goal." Chloe doesn't answer. She's gone, looking out the window, very far away. "What are you thinking right now?" Debi asks gently.

"Nothing." She returns to us. "Do you have a kid?" she asks Debi.

"No, I haven't been able to get pregnant. We're still trying."

"How many pregnant women have you worked with?"

I don't know why Chloe wants to know Debi's credentials, but Debi's not fazed in the least. "I've been a nurse for five years, but have always worked with babies and moms."

"More than a hundred?"

"Oh yes, many more than that."

Debi shows Chloe a picture of the developmental stages of an embryo *in utero* and points out one picture that is close to the stage of her fetus. Chloe studies the picture. "It looks kinda funny, with eyes on the side of the head."

"Well, I'm here if you have any questions. You can call or text me anytime you like. We could go out for a walk sometime, if you'd like."

Chloe looks down and lifts her shirt to take a look at her belly. She prods it, and jabs roughly at it in a few places. "If you poke the baby too hard, will it be born with an indent?"

Debi assures her not, if she's gentle.

"Does it pee in there? And drink that back?" Chloe looks incredulous and disgusted.

"Yes." Debi explains about placenta, umbilical cord. "The baby is getting its food from you. You breathe for your baby. Provide food for the baby."

"If my last period was August 22, what was the date I would have gotten pregnant?"

Now, as we are getting up to leave, questions occur to her.

Debi checks an obstetrical app on her phone and tells Chloe her approximate due date.

"No, I mean, what was the date when we last had sex? What was the day I got pregnant?"

"Roughly two weeks after your last period . . . that's if your periods were regular."

Chloe is doing some backwards calculations in her head and counting off days on her fingers. She smiles, then sighs, happy about a memory of the day of her baby's conception. She points to her drawings on the coffee table. "I wants to be a tattoo artist. I was an apprentice, but I didn't have money for a licence, but the guy let me work there."

"Do you want me to come back for another visit?" Debi asks her. "I won't if you don't want me to. This is voluntary."

"Yes, please come back." Chloe looks on the verge of tears. "I'm lonely," she says.

But she remembers something. "Soon, I won't be alone. I'll have a little friend to keep me company." She lifts her shirt and smiles down at her tummy.

27

MAKING AN IMPACT

"HEY, TILDA, can you work another night shift tonight? We need you."

I worked last night and they told me the news. Richard Thornton-Sharp died. At home. Peacefully. In Jim's arms.

Jim sent me an email, "Richard was truly the love of my life and I can appreciate the fact that I had the most wonderful thirty-three years with someone who I loved and who loved me. I am very fortunate to have had this incredible relationship. Richard was an amazing person and in my heart he is still with me as the journey continues."

"Okay, I'll come in for a twelve-hour night shift," I tell Voula, the nurse in charge who's been scrambling all day to find more nurses for tonight.

Hey, I'm a sucker for being needed and patients need nurses. There's no shortage of patients. If there's a shortage of anything, it's nurses and caregivers.

My journey is over now, and I feel nostalgic for it already. I've sent off my impressive collection of hotel swag – over 100 bottles of shampoo, conditioner, body lotion, and bars of soap – to the 360 Clinic for their clients – a tiny token of appreciation.

There are so many things that still make no sense to me in the hospital, like the waste we create and the excessive use of technology; the restricted visiting hours and the no-pet policy. The fact that patients aren't invited to participate in team rounds about their own care. Why aren't people allowed – no, encouraged – to read their own charts? Why do we have so much computer charting that it takes us away from patient care? Why are there nurses and doctors who don't talk kindly – or at times even courteously – to patients, or who can't find it in themselves to sit down and simply listen to what the patient has to say? Why does a nurse have to call a doctor to get a Tylenol or a laxative for a patient? Why can't patients who are well enough to administer their own meds do so? Why are the people who provide the most care to patients (nurses) and to everyone else, the sickest themselves? Why do hospitals have to be so gloomy, bereft of music and art and beauty? Why do staff walk into patients' rooms without knocking? Why is the food so bad, so unhealthful, often inedible? Why, given all the technological advancements, policies, checks, and double-checks, are medication errors still so frequently made? And why is it so easy to get so busy and distracted that you can completely forget that your patients aren't feeling very well? Why is there so much *waiting* in hospitals, and if you do have to wait, why can't someone come out and tell you why and how much longer you'll still have to wait, and maybe even do it with a smile?

I'll stop here.

I've wondered about these things for years. However, in all of my travels outside of the hospital, in all of my visits to homes, clinics, community centres, I saw patient care that was governed by logic, fairness and common sense, administered with kindness and goodwill – not to mention fiscal responsibility and restraint.

More, please.

I've always chosen to care for the sickest patients, making the assumption that that was where the biggest challenges were, where the need was greatest, and where there was the most excitement. But there are other challenges to face and work to be done that are no less important and every bit as *exciting*.

"So," they'd all asked when I was back at work, "how was it?"

"Good. Very good."

"And are you back now for *good*?"

"For good," I say. "For now, anyway."

It doesn't have to be this or that, either-or; it can be *and*.

Audrey always planned that her home would be her last address until the cemetery. After her brief stay in the hospital, she did come home. Hilda, Virginia, and Audrey's cadre of caregivers, friends, and neighbours came to take care of her, even taking turns staying with her around the clock. Now, though, her care is getting to be more than they can handle and she needs a nursing home. But she seems to have reconciled herself to it because she visited one to inspect it. Soon I receive a few more letters – sunflowers, goldfish, fancy bows, and teacups.

At the nursing home they range from 79 to 102 years young. It's a friendly place, clean and very home-ish. A place where it would be hard to become alone-ish.

Yes, I sold my darling little house and contents. I've never been as popular in my life until now that I'm cleaning out the house . . .

I've always known that everyone's life is a story worth telling. With each letter I received from her, Audrey tried to convince me that this was her last chapter. She's said that from the first letter, in the first phone call, during the first visit. Perhaps that's a good way to live.

But now, a few weeks later, the letters have stopped. *I'll call her when I get a chance*, I tell myself, making a note of it on my mental "To Do list." But before I get around to doing so, a call comes late at night, just after midnight. *Who calls this late? It can only be bad news.*

"Is that Nurse Tilda?" a quavering voice asks.

"Audrey," I gasp. "Are you okay?"

"No. Enough is enough."

"What's wrong?"

"I want you to do me in."

"I can't do that, Audrey, you know that. You sound like there's still life in you."

"No, I'm on the way out. I'm almost dead." I hear the sound of rustling pages of paper and can visualize Audrey's slow fingers turning them. "I have a few questions for you, Tilda Sue." Then Hilda gets on the line and explains that Audrey has a bad cold, is very weak, and can't walk anymore. Hilda has been staying with Audrey at night until she goes into the nursing home.

"When will your book be done? I'm not long for this world and I want to read it before I go."

"It's almost finished."

"I hope I live to read it."

"I hope so, too."

"You always say I should hang on longer. Is that for me, or for your readers? Wouldn't it make a more dramatic ending if I die tragically in the final act of your book?"

"No need, Audrey. You've provided enough drama."

"Won't your readers want to know if I made it to the end of your book? Tell them I did."

"Will do. Oh, and Audrey, you're not dying. You're not there, yet."

"That's good to hear." She pauses. "There'll be no more letters from me, Tilda Sue. That's it."

"It's late, Audrey," I say, longing for my bed.

"This is my last chapter. My book of life has now been completed."

"Yes, Audrey."

"Tilda Sue. Are you listening to me?"

"Yes, Audrey."

A long pause ensues. It's time to say goodnight, and hopefully hang up, when Audrey stops me in my tracks. "I'm glad you were part of my dash."

"Your *dash*? What's that?"

"It's the space in between birth and death, like it will say on my tombstone, 1933–2013. It represents all the important people and events of one's life."

To care and be cared for. Anything can be endured if you have that. A home, too.

Live-streaming allows me to sit at my desk in Toronto and attend the ICN conference in Melbourne, Australia, to watch and listen to Judith who is about to give her acceptance speech to nursing representatives from all over the world. Here it's afternoon but in Australia it's tomorrow – fitting for a person as progressive and forward-thinking as Judith Shamian.

This morning, I received a mass email from her, copied to thousands of other Canadians who care deeply about our health care and that of the world.

"I am now president of the International Council of Nurses," it said simply.

Mention of her appointment is in the front section of the national newspapers and on CBC Radio. I don't imagine many people take much notice, but maybe they should. In fact, it's time they did, because even if a small part of Judith's huge vision comes true, it will improve everyone's life. It won't be easy. Will her strong voice be heard over the dominating ones of political interests, big corporations, and the medical establishment? If anyone can do it, Judith Shamian can.

Looking resplendent in a royal-blue blouse and a burnished-orange blazer, and wearing a chunky artsy necklace, Judith stands on the podium before the world, and greets the assemply in Chinese, Spanish, French, and in her own Hebrew/Hungarian-accented English. She starts off with a surprising announcement.

I dedicate my four years as your president to a woman named Tova. She was my roommate in nursing school. I met Tova at the age of eighteen and it was the start of a lifelong friendship until she died of cancer five years ago. Tova immigrated to Australia and lived here in Melbourne. She worked as a burn unit nurse, a mental health nurse, and then a palliative care nurse. She wasn't the president of an organization. She wasn't a politician or a researcher or a manager or director of anything. She was a nurse who cared for patients, families, and communities in the most knowledgeable way possible. Tova, like millions of nurses around the world, worked to make an impact on the lives of the people they touch.

My commitment to you is to remember the impact nurses have on the lives of people. For the legacy of Tova, I have chosen "impact" as the watchword of my term as your president. In English, *impact* is a noun and a verb, a means and an end. It embodies action and outcome. As nurses, we are here to serve, to make an impact, and to ensure that we can practice the best nursing possible, without risking our lives, safety, and without compromising our family life.

Many countries are dealing with poverty, economic crisis, and lack of access to health care. There are growing concerns about the increase in chronic diseases, mental health, aging populations. Too many decisions are being made without nursing's voice. This is unacceptable, because the only way to make an impact on global health is through nursing knowledge and participation, both at the decision-making tables and in hands-on nursing care, from birth to death and from health promotion, disease prevention, primary, acute, critical, chronic, long-term, home, and palliative care.

. . . a nation's prosperity is enhanced by a strong nursing profession. It is simple: you see, the wealth of our nations depends on the health of people, and the health of people depends on nursing. How we will have an impact? Look around and cast your eyes on this global nursing community. We know how to keep people well, help them heal, and save lives. We can transform illness-focused health care to a wellness-focused one. When we unite as one profession we are a powerful force. We are the *nurses* of the *world*, and we have the potential to make the people of our countries healthier.

She tells them she has 1,460 days to make a difference and that she intends to make use of every single one of them. "Let's get to work," she says. "There's no time to waste."

A few days later, Judith's back in town, and I get one more meeting with her, at her home on the Sabbath. There's no real purpose for this meeting, I just want to congratulate her personally. She's just arrived home from Australia and should be jet-lagged, but doesn't look it in the least. She's fresh and refreshed, younger-looking than I've ever seen her in a loose comfortable dress and silk stockings without shoes. To my delight, I notice that she's had a pedicure, her toenails polished in a pattern of copper, silver, and gold – shiny celebratory colours. Her fingernails are in the same multicoloured pattern. She looks content, the way a person looks, not immediately after crossing the finishing line of a marathon, but a few hours later. Tonight, when three stars appear in the sky and the Sabbath ends, her week will begin and she'll be back to work. In fact, tomorrow she leaves for Europe to attend a conference on health care workers in war-torn countries.

Her husband comes into the room and wishes me a *Shabbat Shalom*, Sabbath Peace. He nods at Judith. He's beaming, busting with pride – *kvelling*, would be the exact Yiddish term. "Are you as proud of her as we are?"

Yes, of course, but even more than proud, I am happy, more hopeful for the world.

And there is something else to celebrate. Good news about VON. The Board and the new corporate leadership are working very hard to turn things around. Restructuring, advanced technological innovations, fiscal restraint, and correcting inefficiencies. I'm not sure what all of that means other than the important bottom line: VON will be saved.

"This beautiful organization will live on," Judith says. "From strength to strength," she murmurs reverently, like she's conferring a blessing.

There's no need for tea or coffee, nor reading or debating. We take up our usual places on the chairs. Is it my imagination or has our relationship shifted? I don't know for sure, but I face her now as a partner, as colleagues. We sit back and take a break from the work that usually occupies us both so intensely. It's far from completed, our goals have not been reached, but it's time to rest. Together we sit, gazing out at the street, the neighbourhood, the city, and the world unfurled before us, the world with all its goodness and all of what still needs repair.

"I like how you mentioned nurses' health and safety, and their family life."

"Yes, I worry about how nurses can maintain their health – and their compassion – and sustain it for an entire career. It's not enough to care for patients. We have to care for nurses, too."

I have to ask. "Was Tova her real name?"

"Yes."

We both know the meaning of that word. *Good.*

It's all good.

Yes.

Postscript

Early this morning, I finished writing this book. I typed the last word – "Yes" – and pushed the Send button to shoot this manuscript off to Elizabeth Kribs, my editor at McClelland & Stewart/Random House Canada.

A little less than an hour later, I received a text from Jean Kilfolyle, Audrey's friend.

"Audrey is in palliative care. She's on oxygen and unresponsive."

It won't be long now, though knowing Audrey, anything is possible.

Around five o'clock this afternoon, Jean called to say Audrey had died.

"She's at peace. She waited for you to finish your book. Thank you for being one of the brightest stars in Audrey's life."

From the first time I met her, Audrey told me she was ready to die. Vivacious and morose, charming and aggravating, generous and stubborn, there were many sides to her, but I never met someone as thoroughly prepared for death and as joyfully engaged in life as Audrey McClenaghan of Kemptville, Ontario.

Safe home, Audrey. Safe home.

Tilda Shalof
October 2013

Acknowledgements

To all who shared their stories, and thus themselves, with me.

Judith Shamian for the opportunity to learn what real *health* – not illness – *care* is all about.

Elizabeth Kribs, Terri Nimmo, and Linda Pruessen at McClelland & Stewart for their superb editing and design.

VON and its staff and volunteers. Special thanks to Owen Adams, Derrick Babin, Darlene Billard-Croucher, Stacey Bourque, Marilyn Chuli, Carol Cooke, Lori Cooper, Krista Dalliday, Maria DesRoches, Suzanne D'Entremont, Joshua Dougherty, Cherie Gilbeault, Sandra Golding, Robert Fraser, Kathy Hardill, Laurianne Hébert, Irene Holubiec, Nicole Hunter, Jon Jewell, Robin Kish, Irena Kesminas, Anne-Renée Landry, Christine LeBlanc, Elizabeth Loftus, Beverlee McIntosh, Janet McLeod, Connie Milliken, Sylvia Mingo, Irene Pasel, Kathryn Roka, Gayle Sadler, Bonnie Schroeder, Judy Stewart, Jan Stutz, Stephanie Vandevenne, Helen Vink, Karen Ursel, Andrew Ward, Joan Wekner, Jackie Wells, and Robert Zwicker.

To VON nurses of Halifax and Yarmouth, Nova Scotia – especially: Josephine Blynn, Frances Brison, Julia Cottreau, Sheila D'Eon, Marg Jenkins, Barb Lutz, Thelma Newell, Ellen Pothier, Barb Rodney – for a rollicking good evening of stories.

Celine D'Gama, Rose Faratro, Anna Gersman, Jennifer Kazmaier and CalaCare Home Health Care, Annie Levitan, Anne Moorhouse; Merilyn Simonds and Jan Walter; Doris Grinspun and the Registered Nurses Association of Ontario; Sandy Zidner, Diane Moretto and Toronto

Public Health; Natalie McLean and Hospice Toronto; Denise Morris and team of the Medical-Surgical Intensive Care Unit, Toronto General Hospital — especially: Stephanie Bedford, Belle Dhillon, Janet Hale, Margaret Herridge, Edna Lee, Kate Mackenzie, Wendy Radovanovic, Janice and Audrey Stanley, Jasna and Jack Tomé and sons.

To the ones who bring me home: Harry, Max, and Ivan Lewis.

You may also be interested in the
following books by bestselling author
Tilda Shalof

NATIONAL BESTSELLER

TILDA SHALOF
A NURSE'S STORY

LIFE, DEATH AND IN-BETWEEN
IN AN INTENSIVE CARE UNIT

With a new foreword by
DR. BRIAN GOLDMAN,
host of CBC Radio's *White Coat, Black Art* and author of *The Secret Language of Doctors*

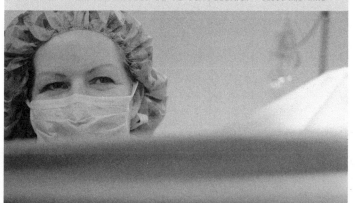

"*GREY'S ANATOMY* SHOULD BE SO COMPELLING." *GLOBE AND MAIL*

THE MAKING
OF A NURSE

AUTHOR OF THE BESTSELLING *A NURSE'S STORY*

TILDA SHALOF

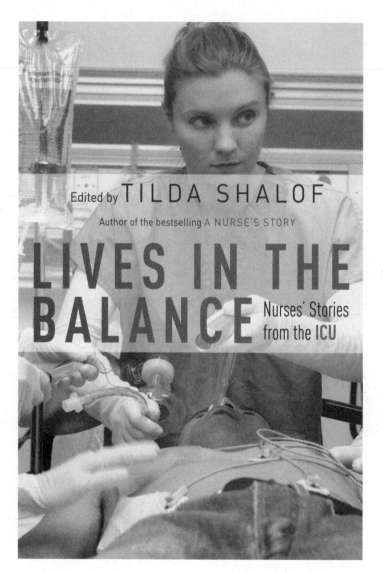

Edited by TILDA SHALOF

Author of the bestselling A NURSE'S STORY

LIVES IN THE
BALANCE

Nurses' Stories
from the ICU

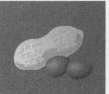

CAMP
NURSE

My Adventures at Summer Camp

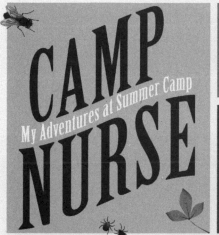

"A rare fly-on-the-infirmary-wall view of a Canadian rite of passage – as well as a postcard of modern childhood." MACLEAN'S

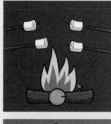

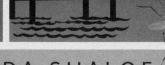

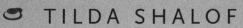

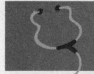

TILDA SHALOF

Bestselling author of A Nurse's Story and The Making of a Nurse

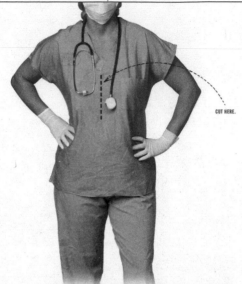

CUT HERE.

"A smart patient knows more about coping with their disease than their physician, and Tilda Shalof's insights into the rigors of heart surgery are even more provocative since she brings a nurse's wisdom to her own operation."

DR. MEHMET OZ, HOST OF *THE DR. OZ SHOW*

OPENING MY HEART

A JOURNEY FROM **NURSE** TO **PATIENT** AND BACK AGAIN

TILDA SHALOF